Dummett

9/25/
8.22A

Joseph Austen Dummett
7 pounds 1 ounce
20½"
Agpar 7.9/10

Dr Chaiken
Dr Lohaus
Howard Co. Gen.
Columbia, Md 21044

9/20/82 Monday
1:45 PM
Dr Chaiken
Dr Valove

Brian Alexander Dummett
7 pounds 4 ounces
18¾"
Apgar 8/9

THE CESAREAN BIRTH EXPERIENCE

the Cesarean birth. experience

A Practical, Comprehensive, and Reassuring

Guide for Parents and Professionals

Bonnie Donovan

with a foreword by
RUTH ALLEN, R.N.C.

and an introduction by
MURIEL SUGARMAN, M.D.

BEACON PRESS : BOSTON

Copyright © 1977 by Bonnie Donovan

Beacon Press books are published under the auspices
of the Unitarian Universalist Association

First published as a Beacon Paperback in 1977
Published simultaneously in Canada by
Fitzhenry & Whiteside Ltd., Toronto

Printed in the United States of America

(hardcover) 9 8 7 6 5 4 3 2 1

Library of Congress Cataloging in Publication Data

Donovan, Bonnie.
    The Cesarean birth experience.
    Bibliography: p.
    Includes index.
    1. Cesarean section.   I. Title.
RG761.D66   618.8′6   76-7742
ISBN 0-8070-2748-0
ISBN 0-8070-2749-9 (pbk.)

A pyramid of love and gratitude to both Billy and Ruth, who helped to make this book a reality.

To Jon and Sarah, two loving and beloved children, who caused this book to be written.

And to Dunnie, with special love.

CONTENTS

ACKNOWLEDGMENTS

Without the assistance, love, and support of two quintessential people, this book quite literally could not and would not have been written.

Ruth Allen, R.N.C., British-trained nurse-midwife, childbirth educator and lecturer, gave technical assistance, hundreds of hours of her time, and her unremitting support. Her well-rounded library of medical texts and journals and childbirth literature was the basis of much of my research. She deserved pages of praise and gratitude, but respecting her modesty, I will simply say: Thank you, dear friend. *Alter ipse amicus.*

Billy helped me find my Muses when I lost track of their whereabouts—and they of mine. He rubbed my back when it hurt from typing all day, stroked my psyche when I felt discouraged, took equal care of the children, and never complained when I kept the light on all night or clacked away at the typewriter at odd hours.

Dr. Muriel Sugarman was especially helpful in making suggestions on several chapters.

Elisabeth Bing, R.P.T., childbirth author and educator, lent valuable assistance.

Valmai Elkins, R.P.T. of Montreal, introduced me to the abdominal tightening exercises which are a boon to cesarean mothers.

Elizabeth Caswell, R.N., and John Caswell, R.N., are to be thanked for the sensitive photographs and their numerous kindnesses.

To Leslie and Fred Hill: thank you for sharing Joshua's birth.

Linda Peterson, friend and class assistant, and Maeva Buckman, R.N., are to be thanked for helping in ways both large and small.

Ruth Rotko and Neil Weisbrod: your efforts were not in vain.

Ann Hutchinson, artist, friend, and true renaissance woman: a rainbow of thanks.

To the people who sent letters and requests for copies of the book (many through ICEA and C/SEC, Inc., who were both most gracious in promoting the book through their newsletters), my gratitude. Your faith in my abilities and intense need for information kept me going when the obstacles seemed greater than I anticipated.

Burleigh Newman: thank you for pointing out the shortcomings in my first drafts.

Bob Goldberg, my attorney: thank you for your legal advice and your kindness and generosity.

To the nurses and doctors of South Shore Hospital, South Weymouth, Massachusetts, who contributed technical information, advice, and support, my deep appreciation. Special thanks to Doctors Gerald Pouliot, Albert Marcus, and James Cox for helping to launch Sarah.

Special thanks to all the others (you know who you are) who supported and encouraged me even when it became apparent that writing this book would take longer than the gestation period of an elephant.

Above all, I should like to express my appreciation to Roberta Fitzsimmons, my editor at Beacon Press, who personifies two essential qualities in an outstanding editor: professional competence and sensitivity to the author and her needs. She started as my editor and became my friend, too.

FOREWORD

At last here is a book for cesarean parents. For far too long the needs of these couples have been neglected. The whole bibliography of childbirth literature ignores this kind of birth experience. All the hows, whys, and wherefores of the cesarean birth have remained veiled in mystery and in profound medical terminology. It seems as though there has been a conspiracy of silence about the subject. Now, at last, it is becoming possible to have a positive birth experience, whether a vaginal or abdominal delivery takes place. Fear of the unknown, and the tensions this fear generates can now be greatly modified. The more aid the parents receive, the more informed and prepared the parents are, the better their birth experience will be, and the more solid the foundation for close bonding between parent and child.

Interest in helping cesarean parents is being expressed in many parts of the country. For example, classes geared specifically to their needs are beginning to be offered. Much more, however, remains to be accomplished. Communication needs to be improved among parents, doctors, childbirth educators, and hospital staff. Many professionals now regard a cesarean delivery as a *purely* surgical procedure, rather than thinking of it in terms of a birth and the advent of a new life. These attitudes will change as more publicity and interest is raised. Information and education in all aspects of the parents' physical and emotional needs must be made available. Parents should share with their obstetricians their feelings about a cesarean experience. Maternity and obstetrical staffs should reassess the way these parents are treated. Are they really included in Family-Centered Maternity Care? Are childbirth educators glossing over the subject in their classes?

As a childbirth educator, I have found that talking with

postpartum couples who delivered by cesarean has been a
learning experience for me. They have been my best teachers.

I have been teaching prepared childbirth classes since 1972.
I became interested in the cesarean delivery when, in one class
alone, five couples delivered this way. Until that time I, like
others, had been glossing over cesarean births. I began doing
some research into the emotional aspects, for many of my
couples had been totally unprepared and were devastated
when an emergency cesarean was necessary. There was no
literature in either America or England. There may have been
a little paragraph about its being an operation, and mention of
Julius Caesar, but that was about all. I began talking to and
corresponding with doctors, nurses, childbirth educators, and
authors. Then in 1974 a catalyst came along in the form of
Bonnie Donovan. She and her husband Bill enrolled in the
regular series, in spite of the fact that they knew their baby
would be delivered by repeat cesarean. From my relationship
with the Donovans, we began to work together on improving
the experience from the parents' point of view. We began
holding informal rap groups with postpartum cesarean parents,
and from these sessions, classes designed to meet the very
special and very different needs of cesarean parents were
initiated at South Shore Hospital. We are now seeing the
results of what we have learned and what we have taught. The
classes, which were started in a totally informal way, have now
developed form, structure, and support from the hospital. Our
graduates now approach the birthday with the knowledge of
what to expect and how to cope, and thus are able to rejoice
in their babies' births. No longer are they passive objects on
whom procedures are performed and for whom everything is
totally new, different, and frightening.

This book is the first step in the right direction. Many,
many more giant strides must be taken in the years to come.

Ruth Allen, R.N.C.
Head Nurse of Labor and Delivery
South Shore Hospital, South Weymouth, Massachusetts

INTRODUCTION

Evidence is rapidly accumulating which indicates that the events which occur in the minutes, hours, and days surrounding the birth of a human infant are critical to the healthy or distorted formation of affectional bonds between the infant and his/her parents and to an enhanced or diminished relationship between the mother and father. As such evidence mounts, thoughtful, concerned consumers and professionals are taking a closer look at medical and cultural interventions into the birth process to assess whether they are truly inevitable, what their positive and/or negative medical effects are, whether there are significant psychosocial consequences, and what the means for minimizing them are.

In a general sense, every intervention into, or complication of, the birth process can destroy or distort the delicate physiological-hormonal-psychic balance programmed into mammalian species through centuries of evolution. Ample evidence exists in zoos and research laboratories all over the world to show that changes in, or interference with, the spontaneous course of pregnancy, birth, or postpartum period in animals can have serious and often fatal consequences for the offspring. Yet not until very recently have humans paused to consider that similar disturbances might be produced even by well-meant interference with, or unavoidable complications of, the human birth process. As an extreme example, we know that there is a striking and significant correlation between prematurity, cesarean birth, or illness resulting in hospitalization during the early weeks of life and the incidence of failure to thrive in infants as well as the incidence of child abuse by parents. Because humans possess consciousness as well as instincts, most parents are able to work out appropriate parental behavior despite obstacles and emotional strain, and most infants born under these circumstances do thrive and do not suffer from child abuse. But, we do not know what more subtle psychological and behavioral effects such events may cause in even the most well-adjusted, most loving parents.

For this reason, the subject of cesarean birth is serious and important. It is a telling indictment of the medical profession (but in a sense it is also a hopeful sign of social growth), that attention to cesarean birth, its consequences, and special needs, had first to come from those parents who had been through a "routine cesarean delivery" and whose feelings of outrage and dismay at the lack of understanding and support they received were channeled into healthy, constructive action.

Cesarean delivery is a lifesaving procedure, and its use has dramatically increased over recent years. While we must be ever on the alert for unnecesary cesarean deliveries as the result of injudicious intervention which upsets the delicate psychophysiological balance of labor, we must also recognize that cesarean delivery is often inevitable if life and mental intactness are to be preserved. Regardless of the reasons for the cesarean delivery, once it becomes necessary for the newborn to reach the outside world through an abdominal incision, certain consequences are set in motion, and every possible means, technique, and mechanism must be brought to bear on the affected family to maximize their comfort and positive experiences and minimize discomfort and negative experiences that might interfere with the rapid formation of those crucial affectional bonds mentioned earlier.

In any life crisis—and birth, especially cesarean birth, is obviously and unarguably a life crisis—factual information has an extremely beneficial effect, and can sometimes mean the difference between an experience that leads to personality disorganization and regression and one which results in greater maturation and integration of the personality. This is not to minimize the importance of other factors such as empathy and support from important human contacts, other extraneous sources of stress, or compensatory activity, but knowledge does promote a sense of choice and control which helps to counteract the feelings of helplessness and hopelessness that accompany unavoidable crises.

This book, *The Cesarean Birth Experience,* provides that crucial factual information as well as suggestions for compensatory activity, for minimizing extraneous stresses, and for seeking support and understanding from human contacts. To my knowledge, it is the first book which has as its primary focus the crisis of cesarean birth, and it is the first to attempt to furnish parents with the tools needed to deal with the crisis.

Being a pragmatist, I must insist that a book alone is not enough. There must be educational classes for parents, more complete training for medical professionals, changes in some deleterious hospital practices, and organized support systems for cesarean families both within the maternity hospital and in the community. In some areas these changes are in progress; in others, they are being woefully neglected. It is in these latter areas that a book such as this can become a catalyst for consumer action and professional cooperation. Being an idealist, I believe it will.

Cesarean birth need not result inevitably in physical or psychological complications. Though accompanied by special stresses, it is, after all, the birth of a new life—a baby—and often, of a family. The concern for life and health that has made a necessary cesarean birth a lifesaving and safe procedure can be directed at making a necessary cesarean birth result in enhanced emotional well-being of the entire family. We now have the knowledge to do both. All that remains is to disseminate and use it.

Muriel Sugarman, M.D.

CHAPTER 1 THE CESAREAN BIRTH

*I*N TERMS OF ANATOMY, the difference between a vaginal delivery and a cesarean section is a matter of a few inches. Yet that difference might just as well be measured in miles when we take into account the quality of the birth experience faced by the majority of the couples whose babies must be delivered surgically.

As recently as 1968, there were only about five cesarean deliveries for every one hundred births. Then, the differences between a vaginal delivery and a cesarean section were not so great. Most mothers were routinely drugged during labor and were unconscious for the birth; there were few prepared childbirth classes available anywhere; fewer books were available for expectant couples; and the role of the father was limited to dropping his wife off at the hospital like a bag of dirty laundry and waiting for a phone call announcing his baby's birth.

Today's climate of concern for pregnant couples is vastly improved. Drugs are used more judiciously in labor and delivery, as both obstetricians and parents have become aware of the dangers of overmedicating women in labor. Childbirth classes given by hospitals, foundations, childbirth associations, or accredited individuals are available in most areas. Many excellent books extol the joys and virtues of "prepared," "Lamaze," "Bradley," "easier," "painless," and "at-home" deliveries. Hospitals now include the father in the birth process. Although many men are dragged unwillingly to the first class or two, most soon become excited about attending prepared childbirth classes, and eagerly anticipate the role they

1

will assume during labor as coach and supporter and during delivery as witness to this very special event.

Family-Centered Maternity Care, which has been implemented in many hospitals, regards the family (mother, father, *and* baby) as a unit rather than as three unconnected individuals. Fathers are considered essential, beneficial, and welcome participants. They are able to cuddle and hold their babies during the hospital stay rather than having to gaze at them through the glass partitions of the nursery window. New mothers are knowledgeable about the advantages of being "aware and awake" for the birth. The new mother may wish to have rooming-in so that the hospital stay becomes a time to acquaint herself with the uniqueness of her baby. Breast-feeding is gaining in popularity.

With the exception of a few areas in the United States and Canada, this glowing picture of childbirth today is accurate— but only with regard to vaginal deliveries. Cesarean parents are the exceptions. They are the "odd" couple for whom almost everything is new, unexpected, different, and frightening.

The need to educate and reassure cesarean parents is greater than ever before. Until recently, there have simply been no classes, books, or films for them; their needs have been neglected and overlooked.

Despite the numerous books on childbirth now available, few discuss the cesarean birth. Those that do, usually limit their discussion to one sentence that tends to go something like this: cesarean section is an obstetrical operation in which the fetus is delivered by means of incisions in the uterus and abdomen.

Because of our understandable lack of knowledge about the cesarean birth, most of us envision a doctor holding a knife over the mother's abdomen, blood gushing all over the place, and possibly a distraught father pacing the waiting room and agonizing as to whether he will have to choose between his baby or his wife.

In 1976 this is myth. The cesarean operation is very safe,

neat, and precise. It is no more gory than a vaginal delivery; in fact, it may be less so. And probably no father will ever have to make a choice. But cesarean parents need and want to know more about the overall experiences of pregnancy, birth, and the postpartum period.

THE GRAPEFRUIT SYNDROME

The cesarean mother, in her dual role as both postoperative *and* maternity patient, has special handicaps. In some hospitals she may be regarded as a "nuisance" because she needs more care and attention than her vaginally delivering counterpart. She may also be labeled as "difficult" or "different" because she does not fit nicely into the category of motherhood as it is supposed to be. She is "The Section in room 204." No one has ever said, "There's a 'vag' down the hall." But there she is, "The Section in room 204." The section? It sounds as though we're talking about a piece of grapefruit!

"Hah! You had your baby the easy way," friends tell the cesarean mother before they launch into tales of their own lengthy, difficult labors and deliveries. Her family may react differently: "Oh, you poor girl. You'll be crippled for life," they say as they wring their hands. Both attitudes are equally incorrect and damaging. There is certainly nothing easy about a cesarean delivery (be it emergency after labor has begun, or an elective or repeat scheduled in advance of labor), nor does it mean that the mother will be an invalid as a result. The truth has been so clouded with myth and misinformation that cesarean parents may not know what to believe.

Most cesarean couples wish that they had been able to find out what happened to them and why. "What went wrong?" some ask. "What did I do that I shouldn't have?" "Why me?" "Why did this have to happen to me?" "What can I do to make the next time better?" Or, "How can I find out what happened, even though I know we'll never have another baby?"

As lifestyles become more casual and childbirth is seen in

more "natural" terms, a great deal of emphasis is placed upon having one's baby with a maximum of understanding and preparation and a minimum of obstetrical management, drugs, and instrumentation. It is a very positive approach to childbirth provided that one's body and one's baby allows for passage through the birth canal in an uncomplicated vaginal delivery. Because the traditional attitude regarding the cesarean delivery emphasizes the surgical rather than the birth aspect, cesarean mothers often feel "left out" and "let down." It is dismaying to hear them refer to themselves as "failures" and natural childbirth "flunkies." This is not the way it has to be.

Fortunately, there is a growing awareness of the need to improve the cesarean birth experience. Individuals, childbirth education associations, and a growing number of doctors, nurses, and support groups have made greater advances in the past two or three years than at any time previously. Articles about the cesarean birth experience are beginning to grace the pages of newspapers and magazines. Childbirth conferences now frequently include cesarean delivery as a topic of information and discussion. Classes have begun in many different locations for expectant cesarean couples. These improvements are not as yet widespread, but pioneers in the field have seen what can be done when an effort is made to prepare cesarean parents through education and emotional support. In other words, the cesarean couple should be regarded in the same way as other parents and families, and be helped to have positive, meaningful, fulfilling birth experiences.

In writing this book, I have been able to draw on my own two cesarean births. The first, which took place in 1969, was so harrowing and traumatic, both physically and emotionally, that I vowed that if I ever had another baby, I would make things different—and above all better. When I became pregnant again in 1973, I assumed that things would have changed, there would be books to read, classes to attend, and films to see. Unfortunately, the atmosphere surrounding the cesarean birth had hardly changed in those five years. And I began to research and write. My early drafts were more subjective than objective. I was unaware then of the depth of my feelings or how necessary and cathartic those early drafts were. Like other cesarean mothers, I had to work through the fears, fantasies, resentments, and unfulfilled expectations that had built up inside me. The result, I hope, is a book that is factual as well as empathetic.

The term "cesarean section," in its numerous spellings and capitalizations, is the medically accurate term for the procedure whereby a baby is delivered surgically instead of vaginally. When necessary for technical accuracy, I use the term "cesarean section." However, when discussing the experience from an emotional and parental point of view, the book's primary objective, I feel that it is much more positive, much more reassuring, and much more to the point to use the words "cesarean birth" and "cesarean delivery" to emphasize the birth rather than the surgery. When we use the words "birth" and "delivery" in relation to the cesarean experience, it serves as a reminder that it is not just another surgical procedure—such as the removal of a tumor—but rather, and most importantly, the birth of a baby. The baby is not an inconsequential side effect of the procedure, he or she is the reason for doing it! I also avoid two other commonly used terms, "c-sec" and "section." They are grating to the ear and tend to reinforce the "Grapefruit Syndrome."

The Grapefruit Syndrome, like the "tension equals fear equals pain" philosophy, is cyclical. It is the cycle of fear, frustration, and stress which resulted from the almost total absence of practical information and reassuring support. Although the physical needs of the cesarean mother and baby have been well met, until recently even the most well-intentioned health care professionals tended to neglect the emotional needs of the cesarean family.

The time is past for cesarean sections. It is now time for cesarean *births*.

CHAPTER 2 INDICATIONS: WHY ME?

WAS IT FATE OR MY FAULT?

*A*N ALL-TOO-FREQUENT reaction to an emergency cesarean is, "Why me? Why did this have to happen to *me?*" Cesarean Parents (mothers, especially) wonder if it was caused by fate or something they did "wrong."

Here are some examples of the emotions experienced by cesarean mothers:

"I couldn't believe that it could happen to me. Not to *me.* We had everything so nicely planned. My husband came to classes and really wanted to help me through labor. But especially we wanted to share the birth of our baby. We wanted to see her arrival together."

"Cesareans happen to *other* women. I did everything right [good prenatal care, proper diet and exercise, reading, attending classes, etc.]. Why did I end up with a section?

"I hated my baby for being too big to come out normally. I despised myself for taking the medication during labor. If only I hadn't done that, maybe I could have avoided having a c-section."

"If only the doctor had let me push longer."

"The nurse was such a witch. She made me get uptight. That's why I had a cesarean. I couldn't stay in touch with my body with her bugging me all the time."

"For some reason I felt that my husband was to blame for all this. I know he wasn't—I really wanted a baby—but I just got so angry with him for putting me through this terrible thing."

"My mother had two sections. She said she almost died both times. More than anything in the world, I wanted to avoid this."

"When the doctor told my husband to leave, because they were going to do a section, I felt both terrified and relieved. I hated having my husband go, he really helped a lot. But another part of me said, 'Thank

God. Thank God. At last it's going to be all over. I won't feel this pain
any more.' "

"All my friends have had babies naturally. One of them even delivered
at home. She said it was the most beautiful time of her life. The others
all had their husbands there for labor and delivery. I was too chicken to
even think about having a baby at home. But we sure looked forward
to having Bob there. He had his camera all ready. We talked for hours at
a time about what it would be like to see our baby born. Sure, I wanted
my baby to be healthy, but I could have killed the doctor when he made
Bob leave me. I was so scared. I didn't think I could face it alone. I
begged the doctor to put me out. I was afraid of the pain. I didn't want
to hear what was happening. Among all the other things I was thinking
about, I kept flashing on the fact that I was going to be *different*. I
wouldn't be able to tell my friends about my baby's birth. I felt cheated.
I was gypped. It wasn't my baby's fault, but I didn't like being left out."

It used to be that when an expectant mother tried to find
out why she had to have a cesarean, she was patted on the
head and told by an avuncular, patronizing obstetrician,
"Now, now, don't worry your pretty little head. Don't ask me
to explain things you cannot possibly understand." Often
parents were content with that answer but, now that people
are more aware of themselves as health care consumers, they
want to know why, what, and even how much the doctor's
services are going to cost. It is important for parents to know
what the indications (medical reasons) for the cesarean are.
Knowing this will help them to deal more effectively and confidently with the situation. It may even help them to achieve
a more positive birth experience or, at least, to view it in a
better perspective.

With few exceptions, it can be said that an emergency
cesarean is a surprise, often to the couple *and* to the doctor.
The expectant woman's pregnancy and early labor may have
been perfectly normal; neither the doctor nor the couple
saw the need for surgical delivery until just a few minutes,
or perhaps a few hours, beforehand. There is usually no reason
to suspect that vaginal delivery will not be possible until labor
has progressed. The couple may have done everything within
their control to ensure the healthy, uncomplicated delivery of

their baby. The mother may have had good prenatal care, eaten the appropriate foods, taken her vitamins regularly, attended classes, practiced her relaxation-breathing techniques, exercised faithfully, gotten as much rest as she needed, and happily awaited the baby's birth. The father may have been just as supportive and helpful as possible. The couple may have read every book they could find on pregnancy and childbirth.

It is not unusual for the early stage of labor to progress in a manner that is unremarkable. Sometimes the doctor informs the couple in advance if s/he thinks the baby may have to be delivered by cesarean; for example, if the baby is in a breech position (see page 12).

The doctor told me weeks in advance that the baby was breech and that if she didn't turn, I might have to have a cesarean. I kept hoping . . . wishing . . . *willing* her to turn. I completely blocked out the thought of a section and concentrated all my efforts on making her turn. I didn't want a section, but my wishful thinking didn't work.

Not all primary (first-time) cesareans are emergencies. There are some indications for performing a first-time cesarean that can be determined in advance. Briefly, some of these indications are diabetes, herpes simplex, chronic illnesses, and pelvic insufficiency (the mother's pelvis is too small to accommodate the passage of a baby).

But the point is that most often, the decision to perform a primary emergency cesarean is not known until labor has advanced. The announcement may be devastating. It may, however, be greeted with relief as well as anguish. If the labor has been especially long, painful, or complicated, the doctor's decision carries the promise that at least something will happen and *soon.*

Boy, was I glad! Labor was just awful. Within minutes after the doctor said he was going to take the baby, they gave me a spinal. Did that feel good! It was instant relief from all the pain. Now that I think about it, I'm not too keen on having to have another cesarean. But I sure didn't mind the first time . . . at least not till it was all over. Then I felt bad.

The couple who have been together for labor are suddenly separated (in most cases). One father, in the days when it was uncommon for the father to wait at the hospital for the birth, much less act as coach and supporter, told me that the doctor telephoned him to ask for his permission to make a little incision. Thinking the doctor meant an episiotomy, the father agreed readily. Hours later, upon arriving at his wife's side, the man was horrified to learn that the "little incision" was a cesarean section. As he said, "If anything had happened to them [his wife and baby], I would have killed myself for not being there."

Another father, told by the medical staff that he would have to wait in the lobby because they were going to "section the baby," thought they were going to cut the baby into pieces. He had heard old wives' tales that babies were sometimes cut to pieces during difficult deliveries. We may laugh at this man's ignorance, but his experience serves as an example of why more information is necessary and why hospitals are sometimes remiss in their responsibility to act as a liaison between the doctor, mother-to-be, and expectant father.

Until recently, most fathers have spent the hour or so it takes to perform a cesarean in waiting rooms and lobbies. They worry, fantasize, and agonize about what is happening to their wives. The mother, meanwhile, is the center of attention —none of it from the person she loves, trusts, and depends upon. One father, who was made to wait in a corridor outside the delivery room, described his experience as follows: "I was really freaked out. That thing [the intercom] kept paging people and in my panic I thought every call was for my wife and baby."

When an emergency cesarean is performed, it may be for one or a combination of reasons. Each case is based upon individual considerations, and takes into account the mother's medical profile. The reasons for a friend's cesarean are not necessarily the same ones for yours.

EMERGENCY INDICATIONS

Fetal Distress. In the past few years it has become common practice to monitor the fetus while the woman is in labor. During labor, and before the membranes—the sac that contains the fetus and the amniotic fluid, also referred to as the "bag of waters"—have ruptured, belts are placed around the woman's abdomen. If the membranes have broken, a tiny electrode may be inserted internally, and attached to the baby's scalp.

Fetal monitors are machines that chart both uterine contractions and fetal heartbeat. These are recorded on a graph continuously. The attending doctor or nurse will read this print-out and interpret it. If a potentially threatening change in the pattern of the fetal heartbeat, an irregularity, and/or prolonged length of contractions occurs, a cesarean delivery may be necessary.

An ominous change in the fetal heartbeat is called fetal distress. It indicates that the supply of oxygen to the baby is endangered and that if labor is allowed to continue, the well-being of the child is jeopardized. The cesarean delivery in such a case is now a relatively safe way out of a potentially dangerous situation. Prior to the introduction of fetal monitoring, the only means of determining the baby's heartbeat in utero was listening, by means of doptones or fetoscopes (the same devices that the doctor may use after about the fifth month of pregnancy during routine visits). They are neither as accurate nor as consistent as fetal monitors. Thus fetal distress is an increasingly more common indication for cesarean delivery as the condition of the fetus can more readily be gauged.

Although there is a great deal of discussion among medical and lay persons about the use, overuse, and/or abuse of fetal monitoring, an unusual change in the baby's heartrate shows that s/he would prefer to be born as quickly and as safely as possible. Opponents fear that the father or hospital staff will become mesmerized by the machine, and watch it, rather than the mother; that the electrode will damage or scar the baby;

that this is a technological invasion of both the mother's body, and the baby's "privacy."

It is important to consider the advantages of fetal monitoring. Indeed, there *may* be a mark left on the baby's head as a result of the placement of the tiny electrode, but it does not endanger the fetus, nor is the mark permanent. The fetus whose systems are overly taxed by the rigors of labor is less likely to have the necessary strength required to cope with the demands of life outside the uterus. He or she will have expended vitally needed energy with the strain of labor. Above all, fetal monitoring can be credited with saving the lives of a number of babies who would not have survived (or who would have experienced difficulties) had labor been allowed to continue and a vaginal delivery attempted.

Cephalopelvic Disproportion (CPD). "Cephalo" refers to the head size of the fetus. When the indication for a cesarean delivery is CPD, it means that this particular baby is too large to pass through the mother's pelvic outlet. Some women are able to deliver ten-pound babies vaginally while others cannot accommodate the birth of a six- or seven-pound baby. Basically, it is a spatial problem. When CPD is the indication, there are two major considerations: one is the structure of the pelvis; the other is the size and/or part of the baby's head that is presented. The pelvis may be small, or formed in an unusual, but not necessarily abnormal, way; or, the baby's head may be flexed so that a larger circumference is presenting, as for example in a brow presentation.

During pregnancy there are three tests that may help the doctor determine if CPD is a potential problem. One test is the X ray, which will show the measurement of the angle and diameters of the mother's pelvis. A second method is pelvimetry, or internal examination of the size of the pelvic outlet by X ray. A third and newer method is ultrasound (sometimes called a "sonargram"), which will show the size and position of the fetus. Even if one or more of these tests indicates a potential problem, the doctor may still allow the mother to go into labor, and she will be watched closely. If there is no progress, or if there are signs of fetal distress, a cesarean will be indicated. However, it is important to emphasize that there may be no reason to suspect CPD until after labor has progressed for some time. CPD is often a "surprise" to both the expectant mother and the obstetrician.

Each woman and each baby are judged on an individual basis. Women who have had one or more vaginal deliveries previously may have CPD in subsequent pregnancies. Although CPD is a frequent indication for a primary cesarean in a woman pregnant for the first time, it can happen to any woman.

Breech Presentation. The ideal, vertex way for a baby to be positioned at the time of birth is with the head facing toward the mother's back and down in the mother's pelvis. An increasingly common indication for a cesarean delivery is breech presentation. A breech birth is one in which the baby wants to come out bottom first (the part usually covered by "breeches").

Not all breech-positioned babies are born by cesarean. Cesarean delivery for breech babies is more common among women who are pregnant for the first time and who thus have an "untested" pelvic outlet. An attempted vaginal delivery of a breech presentation may create the hazards of anoxia (cutting off or reduction of the supply of oxygen to the fetus); premature respiration of the baby before he or she is fully delivered; and/or, there may still be a problem of the head being too large. Imagine that the whole of the baby's body is delivered when it is determined that the head, which is always the largest part of the baby's body, is too large to pass through the birth canal after all. Rather than subject the baby to this dire possibility, a safe, "easy" cesarean delivery is often preferable to a potentially complicated vaginal delivery.

Transverse Lie. The fetus in this position is crossways to the mother's body, with its head and feet almost horizontal to the ground. It is the most dangerous way for a baby to be positioned at the time of birth, for it means that a vaginal delivery

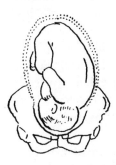 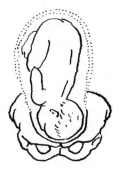 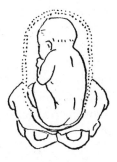

Vertex Presentation   **Brow Presentation**   **Breech Position**

is virtually impossible. Only a tiny or dead baby can be delivered from this position. Anoxia is the major danger although there are others. Transverse lie has always been an indication for cesarean delivery. However, the cesarean delivery is now so safe for both mother and baby that the woman carrying a baby in the transverse position can be reassured that the cesarean delivery is the better, safer, and indeed, *only* way to have her baby.

Dystocia. Dystocia refers to difficult or abnormal labor. Normal labor (eutocia) is: a baby born at full term, presenting head first, within twenty-four hours from the onset of labor, and the process being completed by the natural, unaided efforts of the mother, and without complications.[1] In other words, dystocia is the failure of labor to progress properly, as for instance, when the cervix cannot dilate to the full ten centimeters necessary for vaginal delivery, or when contractions are erratic, nonprogressive, or fail to continue. Dystocia can thus be an indication for cesarean delivery.

Abruptio Placenta. The placenta is the life-support organ for the fetus that is attached to the wall of the uterus. Its function is to sustain and nourish the fetus during gestation. Normally the placenta remains attached to the wall of the uterus and is delivered after the baby. As the name implies, abruptio placenta is the abrupt, usually partial, detachment of the placenta from the uterine wall. It is cause for immediate delivery. There may be abdominal pain or vaginal bleeding. (Note: Any bleeding during pregnancy should be immediately reported to the doctor.)

Placenta Previa. Placenta previa means that the placenta is partially or completely covering the opening of the cervix, and thus endangering the baby's safe exit. There are usually some warning signs such as episodes of painless bleeding ranging from mild to severe during the second and third trimesters of pregnancy. Some doctors prefer to give the fetus the benefits of additional gestational maturation and growth, and will allow the pregnancy to continue for as long as possible under safe conditions for the baby.

Both placenta previa and abruptio placenta are potentially dangerous situations that may be circumvented by cesarean delivery.

Prolapsed Cord. When the umbilical cord slips down before the presenting part of the baby, it is said to be prolapsed. If the cord is prolapsed during labor it will be pinched between the head or the breech of the fetus and the pelvis with each contraction. To avoid further compression and to diminish the dangers of anoxia, a nurse or doctor will hold the fetus up off the cord until the baby can be safely delivered by cesarean. A prolapsed cord can be determined during labor by vaginal examination.

ELECTIVE AND REPEAT CESAREAN INDICATIONS

An elective cesarean delivery means that the indication for the cesarean is known in advance of labor. An elective cesarean may be a primary or a repeat cesarean. A repeat cesarean is just that: a subsequent cesarean delivery. The terms are almost but not quite interchangeable: not all elective cesareans are repeats, although almost all repeat cesareans are elective; unless labor occurs spontaneously or there are other medical factors involved, the repeat cesarean mother will be scheduled for an elective cesarean.

Herpes Simplex. Herpes simplex is a viral infection that may be transmitted to the baby as she passes through the birth canal. Rather than risk possible contamination, a cesarean delivery is indicated.

Diabetes, Renal Disease, Eclampsia, Toxemia. These conditions may be reasons for cesarean delivery of the baby. A scheduled cesarean birth has the advantages of delivering the baby at a time that is optimal for *both* the mother and her baby.

Postmaturity. When a woman has not gone into labor spontaneously approximately two weeks after the estimated date of delivery, the baby may be postmature (overdue). A trial labor may be tried first by means of intravenous introduction of pitocin, a hormone that will stimulate contractions. If labor progresses steadily, and there are no signs of fetal distress, a vaginal delivery will be attempted. A cesarean will be performed if either the baby or the labor warrants it.

The potential danger with postmaturity is that the placenta may begin to dysfunction, creating a hazard for the baby. The placenta is designed by nature to function only for a certain period of time (those *Guinness Book of World Records* pregnancies notwithstanding).

Being two or more weeks overdue, however, does not necessarily indicate postmaturity. The date of conception and thus the due date could be inaccurate. Also, there is usually some leeway with the average gestational period. When in doubt, the obstetrician is the best judge of how "late" the mother is. The doctor may order tests to determine the maturity and well-being of the fetus (see Chapter 5 on tests to determine fetal maturity and well-being).

Previous Cesarean Delivery. In this country the most

common indication for a repeat cesarean birth is a history of previous surgical delivery. Most American doctors adhere to the adage, "once a cesarean, always a cesarean." Their major concern is uterine rupture. It is rare—estimates vary from 1 percent to less than 1 percent—but it is a catastrophe that would result in certain death of the fetus, and could possibly jeopardize the mother's life. In addition, the mother may encounter the same problems she experienced with the previous delivery. For example, if she had difficulty in giving birth vaginally to a 7-pound baby because of cephalopelvic disproportion, it is likely that a CPD problem might arise with this delivery. A subsequent vaginal delivery is possible. The question is: is it preferable? A discussion of the advantages and disadvantages of subsequent vaginal delivery is found in Chapter 6.

Unusual Indications. The mother who has an unusual medical condition will be made aware of it by her obstetrician, and should turn to her doctor for explanations and answers to her questions. Unusual indications include: tumors—such as cervical, fibroid, or ovarian cysts—which would block the birth canal exit; preeclampsia in women pregnant for the first time for whom the usual therapy has not worked; occasionally, chronic heart disease (it has been speculated that women with heart conditions often have rapid, fairly easy labors as "nature's compensation" for their condition); a hysterectomy that is to be performed concurrently; and, increasingly more common, in cases where women have lost babies following difficult labors.

When the decision is made to do a cesarean delivery, it is important to remember that there are a number of factors to be taken into account. Each pregnancy, each mother, and each baby are different. The indications are always judged on an individual basis, taking into account the mother's medical history, the progress of contractions, dilation of the cervix, possible signs of fetal distress, and other conditions that make it necessary to deliver the baby as quickly and safely as possible.]

If your baby is to be delivered by cesarean, it is important to bear in mind that you are *not* a failure. There is everything *right* about ensuring a child the safest, easiest, best possible delivery. Having a baby is not a challenge to your femininity, nor is it a game of Russian roulette. A healthy baby and a positive birth experience for the family are the most important considerations.]

[Cesarean childbirth has advantages which far outweigh the possible disadvantages. The most important advantage is that the cesarean delivery may improve your baby's chances of viability (survival), and reduce the likelihood of learning disabilities, mental retardation, brain damage, or certain physical handicaps. Why subject any baby to possible problems when they can be effectively avoided? For a scheduled cesarean birth, the elimination of the discomforts of labor may be welcome. The newborn cesarean baby, who has not had her head molded from passing through the birth canal, may be initially more attractive. (The heads of vaginally delivered babies do not stay molded or misshapen for long, but this is one minor advantage to the cesarean delivery.) Cesarean babies may have higher Apgar ratings (see page 100) than they would have if they had been put through a strenuous or difficult vaginal delivery. Parents who have older children at home may appreciate being able to know at least a day in advance when the new baby will arrive so they can make preparations for the care of the older children (and pets and houseplants, too). Fathers who wish to take time off to help out with the new baby have a better idea of when to ask for vacation time. Mothers sometimes look forward to having an afternoon to themselves (albeit in the hospital).]

[As recently as forty or fifty years ago, the prospect of survival for the cesarean mother and baby were slim. Tremendous strides have been made that ensure the survival of both mother and <u>baby</u>, as well as give cesarean babies an often better opportunity to thrive than they might have had under adverse vaginal birthing conditions. An "easy" (that is, uncomplicated and safe) cesarean birth is preferable to a long, hard, or difficult vaginal delivery.

Parents who anticipated a beautiful, shared birth experience, and who are confronted with an emergency cesarean delivery should not feel ashamed because they have failed. Instead, they should reassure themselves that their plans were not in vain. Having a baby by cesarean delivery is often a way to have the best of both worlds: a healthy baby and a joyous occasion for the parents.

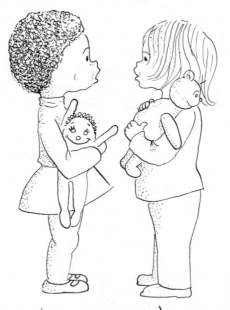

YOU'RE A UNITARIAN? I'M A CESAREAN!

THE CESAREAN MOTHER: WHO IS SHE?

The classic image of a "typical"cesarean woman is that of a
short, small-boned, perhaps frail, nervous creature. Tiny feet
are supposed to be another way to spot the woman who will
have to deliver by cesarean. Some people say that a pointed
jaw, or thin lips betray the woman who must have cesarean
delivery. All elderly primigravidas (women having their first
child after the age of thirty) are supposed to need cesarean
delivery. Just as women who have irregular, painful periods are
blamed for bringing them on themselves, so too, it is whis-
pered, women who are uncomfortable in their roles as child-
bearers are to blame for imposing cesarean deliveries upon
themselves.

The only generalization that can be made about the
"typical" cesarean woman is that she comes in all sizes, shapes,
ages, and from every ethnic and socioeconomic background.
With new, sophisticated tests of fetal maturity and well-being,
and because the cesarean procedure is now a safe alternative
to a complicated lying-in, the number of cesareans is rising.
Along with this increase, the kinds of women who have
cesarean births have come to include almost any childbearer—
even mothers who have had one or more vaginal deliveries.

There is nothing "abnormal" or "wrong" with the cesarean
woman. Women who are almost six feet tall may sometimes
require an abdominal delivery. Happy, feminine women who
produce many children by choice may need to deliver by this
alternative means. Socialites, welfare recipients, single
mothers, career women, factory workers, doctoral candidates,
eighth grade drop-outs—anyone may need a cesarean. The
classic image of the woman who delivers by cesarean has come
to be less a matter of the mother's physique than of the baby's
position, general condition, or gestational maturation.

If all women under five feet tall had to have cesareans, there
would be no other way of giving birth in countries such as
India, Pakistan, China, and Japan where almost all the women
are short by American standards. In those countries, women

who are over five feet tall are often considered unusually tall. This is not to say that American women under five feet tall are excluded from the list of those who have cesarean deliveries. An early 60's study reported in a medical journal indicated that of 117 women under 5 feet, a slightly higher percentage did have cesarean births. The point is that the cesarean mother is anyone.

CHAPTER 3 PREGNANCY

*A*LMOST WITHOUT exception the cesarean pregnancy progresses in much the same way as the pregnancies of women who deliver vaginally. The cesarean mother experiences the same anticipations, joys, trepidations, and physical sensations shared by others. Questions common to all expectant couples arise: Will our baby be all right? Will pregnancy and birth affect our relationship? Will we be able to do the same things we used to? How can we support a family financially?

Pregnancy is a time of emotional ambivalence. The pregnant woman is very vulnerable. She experiences mood swings that confound her. She may be ecstatic about the baby growing inside of her most of the time. At other times, she may tearfully wonder why she thought getting pregnant was a good idea in the first place. Not only does the body change, but the hormonal balance is shifted so that pregnant women sometimes feel as though they are on an emotional roller coaster. One minute they are as happy as clams; the next, they may be in tears over the most trivial incident. Physical changes put her off balance, too, both literally and figuratively. When a woman is pregnant, she is pregnant from the ends of her hair to the tips of her toes. Her whole body, not just the contents of her uterus, is involved. Those around her may find the changes as bewildering and hard to deal with as she does. Within seconds she can change from "benevolent earth mother" to "wicked witch." At times when she needs support and reassurance most, her attitudes may make it difficult for those around her to give it. Pregnant women can be likened to porcupines: they're soft, loving, and in need of cuddling on the inside, but occasionally present an exterior that makes it hard for their families to get close. Pregnancy is a tumultuous occasion. The "couple" become a family. The woman is to become a mother, and may feel that she has lost her "girlishness." Now is the time when she must "grow up," no matter how young or old she is when she has her first baby. Her relationships with the baby's father and future grandparents also change. The parents' greatest hopes and deepest fears come to the surface. Pregnancy and childbirth have social, economic, sexual, and individual implications. With so much to think about, pregnancy may be a time of stress for the couple, especially the mother, even if the baby is wanted and planned for.

The Role of the Father. Being the father of a baby who decides to come into the world by cesarean alters the father's role—but only slightly. During pregnancy the cesarean father will do the same things as any other expectant father: support his wife emotionally, attend prenatal visits to the obstetrician when possible, rub his wife's back, pitch in with the chores, help ready the baby's room and equipment, and participate in prenatal classes. Unless labor occurs spontaneously, the elective cesarean father will know in advance when the delivery is scheduled, which will enable him to make plans so he can spend as much time as possible with his wife and baby in the hospital and during the first week or two at home.

Because the newly delivered cesarean mother must have additional help, the father will play a key role in helping the family achieve the best possible start.

COPING WITH PHYSICAL DISCOMFORT

A number of minor but disconcerting conditions are associated with pregnancy. What can be done to relieve these problems?

Here are some suggestions which may be helpful:

Heartburn. As the uterus grows, the entrance to the stomach can get pushed into the chest cavity, and this may cause heartburn. Instead of three big meals per day, try eating a number of small meals. Stuffing oneself with quantities of food at any one sitting will only aggravate the problem. Junk foods and fried or fatty foods will also increase the chances of heartburn. It is better to stand up or sit up for a while after eating. Reclining may make the condition worse.

Hot Flashes. During pregnancy there will be two extra pints of blood in the body, most of which is in the uterus. When a body is too hot, cool it off. Warmish baths are good. Turning down the thermostat will save energy as well as keeping the body cooler. If you feel comfortable, take your clothes off. If not, try wearing loose cotton garments. Underpants are unnecessary and may, if synthetic, increase the likelihood of vaginal infection—a condition to which pregnant women are prone. Cotton allows the skin to breathe. Rayon and other synthetics and blends do not allow for the free exchange of air. Bras can be discarded, too, unless the breasts are enlarged or uncomfortable.

Chest or Rib Pains. Pain or discomfort under the ribs or chest should be brought to your doctor's attention. (It is always a good idea to write down questions for the doctor when they come to mind. Keeping a special notebook handy is better than saving questions in your head. Unless you write them down as you think of them, you'll probably forget most of them when you are in the doctor's office). Pressure is probably caused by the fact that as the baby grows the chest expands sideways and some organs get pushed out of place. Some babies learn early that their mother's ribs are excellent for kicking and nudging. To cope, place your arms above your head and stretch out to the opposite side from where you're being kicked. Or, raise both hands over your head and reach for the sky.

Poor Circulation. Blood flows from the head, to the heart, to the baby, and finally to the feet. As it returns it has a harder time getting back up. Elevate your feet on a pillow several times a day and at night to improve circulation.

Shortness of Breath. When a pregnant woman lies flat on her back, she invites shortness of breath because the weight of the uterus and baby are on the *vena cava,* the major vein going into the heart from the lower extremities. Lying flat on the back may also reduce the amount of oxygen mother and baby receive. As a general rule, never let the baby lie on you. It is permissible for you to lie on the baby. Women who never felt the urge to lie directly on their stomachs often crave sleeping this way during pregnancy. Go ahead if you want to: it won't hurt the baby, but it may be uncomfortable for you. Some women place twin beds together with a space in between just wide enough to accommodate their bellies. The head, shoulders, and chest are on one bed, and the legs and feet on another. Another (perhaps better) solution is to place a stack of pillows under your chest and hips. A foam block scooped out in the middle may also allow you to lie comfortably on your stomach. The best position is to lie on your *left* side, with pillows under your shoulders and between your legs, which should be slightly flexed at the knees.

How Much To Eat. The rule is to *eat for one and drink for two.* The best diet does not necessarily include extra calories (unless you are underweight), but meaningful calories. Adhere to the dictum, "Don't count calories but make each calorie count."

Extra fluid *is* necessary. Pure fruit juices are preferable to drinks which are primarily sugar and water. Water is a good thirst-quencher and does not have any calories at all. Milk, cocoa, shakes, tea or coffee, or even beer or wine are superior to soda pops and sugared drinks. (Note: avoid too much caffeine).

Leg Cramps. Cramping of the legs and feet is probably due to the hormone progesterone secreted by the ovaries to soften the pelvic ligaments, and your leg ligaments can be affected, too. To relieve cramps in the legs or feet, place your feet against a wall or the end of the bed and push for a few seconds several times. If someone is there to help you, ask the person to hold your foot and firmly press your toes toward your head until the cramp is relieved.

Extra Pigmentation. Patches of dark skin on the body, and a line extending from the navel to the pelvic bone are fairly common during pregnancy. There is little that can be done, but this extra pigmentation will clear up after the baby has been born. This extra coloration may serve to "toughen" the body in preparation for labor. If you are a repeat cesarean mother, remember that your body doesn't know it won't have to go through labor.

Stretch Marks. Either you get them or you don't. If your body is prone to stretch marks, you will get them no matter what you do. A good diet and exercise will help prevent them. Tight clothing may aggravate the condition. Baby oil is inexpensive and works as well as expensive creams and lotions —no matter what the advertisements claim. Use it in place of a makeup remover, bath oil, or as massage oil. It might even help those stretch marks a bit. Vitamins E and A may also help prevent stretch marks and dry skin. During pregnancy, it is best to check with your doctor before taking additional amounts of these or any other vitamin or mineral supplements.

Sexuality. Some women discover that they are aroused more easily during pregnancy. Partially, it may be caused by hormonal changes, and perhaps in part to the new awareness and pride a woman may have in her changing body. Making love may seem freer and less complicated during pregnancy, since birth control is unnecessary. Unless there are special medical conditions, pregnant women can do anything they like in the way of making love. Always check with your doctor if you have questions. Few doctors now impose bans on intercourse during the first three months and the last six weeks of pregnancy (except in special cases).

The mother may want and need the expression of love during this time, and the father has the same needs and drives as ever. As the baby grows the couple may discover that the "missionary" position of lovemaking is uncomfortable—especially for the mother. Pregnancy can be a time of exploration and experimentation with different positions, oral sex, and pleasuring which includes or excludes penetration. The mother-to-be may enjoy the closeness and relaxation that lovemaking brings, but she may find that she does not always have to achieve orgasm to be fulfilled.

There are women who are "turned off" to lovemaking during pregnancy. It may be an excuse to keep her husband from "bothering" her. More commonly, however, it is the extra physical fatigue, the discomfort of the enlarged uterus, intermittent nausea, and other physical problems. Or, the mother may truly fear that making love will somehow damage or hurt the baby, especially if she has had a miscarriage or stillbirth. As always, she should check with her doctor.

Backache. Pregnant women are subject to backaches for two reasons: (1) that human beings have evolved into creatures who stand on two feet, rather than walking on four legs, and (2) that our machine age has eliminated almost totally tasks that required exercise. Backache will not be as frequent a problem if you stand up straight, tuck your fanny in (imagine that you are carrying a cork around in your bottom and you don't want it to fall out), and keep your shoulders back. Exercise and lifting properly by kneeling instead of bending from the waist also help.

Tailor Sitting. Sit on the floor with your legs crossed at the ankles in a position similar to the yoga lotus position. Allow your shoulders to be slightly relaxed. This exercise helps to distribute the weight of the pregnant uterus in a more comfortable manner. It also promotes muscle tone in the pelvis and thighs.

Pelvic Rock. The pelvic rock will help relieve backache and promote muscle tone. It can be done standing or resting on your hands and knees on the floor.

To do the pelvic rock standing up, place one hand on your abdomen just below the bulge and the other hand on your lower back. Push your pelvis forward. Count slowly to three. Then push the pelvis back and hold to the count of three. Do several times each day or whenever you have a backache.

The pelvic rock can be even more effective if you get down on your hands and knees either on the floor or on a firm bed. Push the pelvis forward, count slowly to three, and then arch only your hips and lower back, again counting to three. Often the relief will be immediate.

Pelvic-Floor Exercises. Maintaining muscle tone in the pelvic-floor area is important not only during pregnancy but throughout your adult life. The pelvic floor is the series of elastic muscles used in defecation, urination, and intercourse. They also support the uterus and fetus. If muscle tone is not maintained, a prolapsed uterus can be the result and can cause backache or extreme pain. Lack of muscle tone can also lead to difficulty in muscle coordination during urination or defecation. Men are surprised to learn that they, too, have pelvic floor muscles; if their muscles become lax, they may suffer from prostate and other problems.

Two exercises should be practiced daily. One is to imagine that you are holding a pencil in your vagina and "write" the numbers from 0 to 9 with the pencil. The second exercise is to pretend that your pelvic floor muscles have become an elevator. Start at the first floor, then bring the elevator up to the second floor, and hold there to the count of 10. Bring the elevator up to the third, fourth, and fifth floors, stopping at each floor long enough to count to 10. Reverse the process until you are back on the first floor. Instead of stopping, plunge the elevator down one more floor into the basement. To complete the exercise, bring the elevator back up to the first floor and relax.

These exercises can be done inconspicuously any time during the day. Some people do them while cleaning the house, watching television, sitting in the car waiting for a light to change, or wherever. They should be practiced several times a day. You may feel "clumsy" or "uncoordinated" when you first begin. With practice comes proficiency. In addition to promoting muscle tone, these exercises can be a boon to your sex life. Try them the next time you make love. If you haven't done them before, they will add an extra, interesting dimension to your lovemaking.

Drugs. Until the horrible thalidomide scandal of the early 60's, the medical community assumed that the placenta ". . . was a sort of guardian angel, a St. Peter standing at the gates of the umbilical cord to let needed nutrients through while holding back harmful germs and chemicals. [German measles was one known exception] . . . Rather than being a barrier to the transfer of drugs from the mother to the fetus, writes Dr. Virginia Apgar of the National Foundation-March of Dimes, 'the placenta is a sieve. Almost everything ingested by or injected into the mother can be expected to reach the fetus within a few minutes.' Alcohol, antibiotics, aspirins, barbiturates, sulfonamides and tranquilizers are but a few of the common, and possibly harmful, substances known to get through."[1] Katharine Milinaire in *Birth* further cautions that,

This includes harmful chemicals, soda pops, . . . or puffing any kind of smoke as a daily habit. . . . Most of the damage that occurs because of drugs happens during the first four months of pregnancy. At that time some damage can occur to the baby's growth because the cells are being formed and the structure of the new person is developing. In later months, drugs could cause minor complications. The problem is that most women, even though they may know of their pregnancy during the early months, do not realize the extent of damage that can be caused by drugs. This is especially true at this early stage since you do not really feel or look pregnant. Yet it cannot be overemphasized that these are the most crucial months in the formation of the new being.[2]

Common sense and a wealth of easily obtainable information tells us that drugs—either prescription or over-the-counter—should be used only with the advice and consent of your obstetrician.

It is now acceptable in all but a few social and religious circles to drink. Will the *moderate* use of alcohol during pregnancy adversely affect the unborn baby? Probably not. In fact, a glass or two of wine with dinner may serve to relax the mother-to-be. Warm milk or a nightcap before bed may also help you to fall asleep. (Alcohol is now given intravenously in some cases of premature labor to stop contractions.)

By our own government's estimate, at least eighteen million people have tried marijuana. It stands to reason that among these millions, a few have been female and pregnant. What is the truth about marijuana and its effects on the fetus? No one knows the answer. You may have friends who have had perfectly healthy babies even though they smoke marijuana regularly, but no drug (including tobacco) is without potential danger to the consumer and the developing fetus.

Women who smoke marijuana or do any other kind of drug (uppers, downers, cocaine, LSD, etc.) should probably talk with their doctors. Usually there is some hesitation because the expectant mother fears that the doctor will not understand, will disapprove, or will compound her guilt by telling her she will almost certainly give birth to a deformed or damaged baby. If you simply must smoke during pregnancy (either marijuana or cigarettes), or if you take any other kind of drug, bear in mind that all drugs in all quantities may have an adverse effect on you and your unborn baby. If you cannot give up your indulgences, it may be helpful if you keep the indulgence to a bare minimum, scrupulously maintain a well-balanced diet, take prenatal vitamins regularly, and get adequate rest and exercise. One of the problems is that drugs deplete the body's supply of essential nutrients and create an additional drain on energy reserves and the body's ability to avoid or fight infection.

In cases of emergency, or if you would like to wean yourself from any kind of drug, medical advice and/or counseling are beneficial. Telling the doctor that you smoke dope (or take drugs) probably won't be the first time the doctor has encountered the situation—and it won't be the last. If your own doctor makes you too uncomfortable, try calling a clinic or "hot line." They will be able to put you in touch with someone who specializes in drugs.

Feeling guilty and spending hours of worrying about having had eight drinks at the last cook-out, smoking a pack of cigarettes a day, or indulging in an occasional joint will probably have a more deleterious effect than the act itself. It is better to say, "I did something I shouldn't have. I'll try not to do it again."

A pregnant woman has the choice of what goes into her body. The baby doesn't. Before drinking quantities of soda pop, smoking cigarettes, or having a joint, ask yourself, "Am I willing to take a chance with the health and well-being of my baby?"

Diet. The importance of a "good" diet during pregnancy is universally accepted. For the cesarean mother, it is even more important. The physical stress of the cesarean delivery (that is, surgery, anesthesia, medications) will deplete vitamins and minerals excessively (although temporarily). After the baby is born, the mother's body will be extremely taxed in caring for her newborn, and coping with the regular household chores.

This book does not attempt to explore diet and nutrition in depth, because there are numerous books on the subject. *Let's Have Healthy Children* and *Let's Get Well* by Adele Davis; *Back to Eden,* by Jethro Kloss, and *The Complete Handbook of Nutrition* by Gary and Steve Null are but a few of the many fine books that thoroughly cover the subject of nutrition. Agricultural extension agencies and the U.S. Government Printing Office are excellent sources of inexpensive, informative material on diet and food preparation.

We all know what is proper nutritionally—but what we *should* be eating does not always coincide with what we actually put into our bodies. A general rule to follow is to include foods from each food group daily (protein, vegetables, fruits, grains) and to eat foods as close to the way nature made them as possible (and palatable). Most obstetricians routinely prescribe prenatal vitamins as a supplement and safeguard. It is a good idea to take them faithfully even if your diet is excellent. If you prefer organic or natural vitamins to the ones prescribed by your doctor, ask for a sample of the prescribed brand (provided to the doctor free by the manufacturer). Coordinate the dosage of vitamins and minerals in the prescription tablets to organic vitamin supplements. You will probably have to take more than one capsule, but the effort is worthwhile if you prefer nonchemical preparations, because organic vitamins and minerals may be more easily assimilated.

The following are some suggestions made by pregnant women. You may find them helpful and a welcome variation to your usual diet:

Nibbles and Snacks. Instead of the usual "junk" foods, the following are nutritious and delicious:

raisins

unsalted nuts

yogurt (make your own flavored kind at a lower price than the individual containers by purchasing a quart of plain, unflavored yogurt; then add honey, wheat germ, jam, fresh fruit, etc.)

fresh fruit

raw vegetables with or without a dip (eating lots of raw vegetables and fruit will help prevent constipation)

cottage cheese

cheese (the natural varieties such as cheddar or swiss, rather than the processed type such as Velveeta) with or without wholewheat or whole-grain crackers

oatmeal bread with honey

a peanut butter and honey sandwich

super shakes (milk blended with ice cream and/or

bananas and/or a raw egg and/or chocolate and/or
vanilla extract and/or strawberries—quick, light, and
easy to digest)

cereal and milk and fruit (toasted wheat germ, honey and
fruit is great!)

predigested liquid protein (available at health food stores
and a quick pick-me-up)

shrimp cocktail (if you can afford it)

an avocado and sprout sandwich

chef salad (an anything-goes combination such as lettuce,
shredded cabbage, carrots, grated cheese, sliced or
diced leftover meat, raisins, sunflower seeds, raw or
cooked and chilled cauliflower or broccoli, grated or
sliced zucchini or summer squash, sprouts, croutons,
avocado slices, artichoke hearts, boiled eggs, etc.)

Some other things to keep in mind:
Breakfast is the most important meal of the day. Your body
has been without food for many hours and needs to be
nourished. If morning sickness occurs in early pregnancy, it's
okay to delay breakfast. Eat as soon as you feel able to. If
you skip breakfast, you'll be tired and dragged out—and you
may even become dizzy.

Bake your own bread if you have the time and inclination—
and use wholewheat flour or add soya granules, nonfat dry
milk, or wheat germ to give your baked goods, (bread, muffins,
rolls, cakes, or cookies) additional nutritive value. If you must
rely on store-bought bread, think about buying oatmeal,
wholewheat, or whole-grain varieties. Most soft commercial
white breads have had nutrients and fiber removed in pro-
cessing.

Keep your consumption of sugar to a minimum. Sugar is
caloric and non-nutritive, and it is not easily assimilated. For
sweeteners, use honey, maple syrup, or molasses as much as
possible in coffee and tea and on toast.

To avoid constipation and hemorrhoids (a malady frequently occurring during pregnancy), eat lots of fiber foods,

fresh vegetables, fruits, and foods rich in vitamin B complex (yeast, liver, whole grain cereals).

Eating well, obtaining adequate rest, exercising, and abstaining from drugs is essential for your baby's growth and development and to supply yourself with the resources needed to keep fit and well. If you have maintained an adequate diet during pregnancy, when the time comes for you to have your baby, your body will have a storehouse of vitamins and minerals on which to draw. Some vitamins, such as vitamin C, are rapidly depleted and must be replenished daily. If you feel physically well during pregnancy, you will be able to cope more effectively with caring for the baby and seeing yourself through the postpartum period. Good nutrition is an insurance policy for both the unborn baby and the mother.

Your diet should not undergo a drastic change during pregnancy (unless your obstetrician has special reasons for insisting that you stick to a prescribed diet), although pregnancy is often a good time to gradually introduce new foods to yourself and your family. And, don't be a martyr *all* the time. Treat yourself and your family to occasional "splurges." We all need positive strokes (rewards) sometimes.

Your pregnant body will place extra demands upon you. Prenatal vitamins and minerals will supplement your diet, but they should not be relied on as replacements for any foods— especially raw fruits and vegetables. Feeling well during pregnancy will make the potential stress of an operative delivery less taxing, and will probably decrease the amount of time it takes you to recover fully. The demands of pregnancy, surgery, childbirth, and childcare are great. All pregnant women, and especially cesarean mothers, are well advised to provide themselves with adequate resources to cope happily and healthily.

EXERCISE

Exercise (combined with a good diet) is the best insurance policy a pregnant woman can have. Like a health plan or life insurance, it pays regular dividends from the very first day; and you can "borrow" against it when you need it during pregnancy, childbirth, and later when you are recuperating.

Why should a woman who is to deliver by cesarean need any exercise? After all, she probably won't have to prepare herself for the rigors of labor– right? True, labor is usually forestalled in elective and repeat cesareans by scheduling the delivery in advance of the due date. Getting into, or staying in, shape during pregnancy is important to speed up the recovery process. If you have your baby in a state of fitness (fitness does not mean bulging muscles), you will be better able to care for yourself and your baby. Your figure will return more quickly—and getting back into shape soon after delivery will be good for your soul as well as your body.

The easiest, cheapest, and most convenient form of exercise during pregnancy is walking. The fresh air is good for you and supplies added oxygen to your baby. Walking will make the strains of carrying around almost twenty extra pounds easier. It also promotes relaxation and muscle tone. If you are in shape during pregnancy, the delivery may go easier for you, and it will make those first few days and weeks after the baby is born more comfortable.

Unless you were a physical fitness aficionada before pregnancy, the thought of daily exercise at this time may be less than welcome. You may feel too tired, too big, too. . . . But as an expectant mother you have one really positive thing going for you: motivation. Most pregnant women are highly motivated to ensure the best possible start for their babies. This includes diet, prenatal visits, vitamins, and exercise.

No exercise program should begin with a vigorous workout one day and sore muscles the next. You won't want to continue. Before beginning any exercise program, check with your doctor. Always begin slowly and build up.

Any exercise regularly undertaken before pregnancy can usually be continued during pregnancy. If you swam, rode horseback, or played tennis daily, you will probably be allowed to continue—but check with your doctor first. A few sports are prohibited and dangerous during pregnancy—such as scuba diving, skydiving, and water-skiing.

Whatever exercise you do, pursue it on a regular basis. Try to make it interesting and enjoyable. Yoga is one example of an exercise that combines discipline of the mind with that of the body. It is also a superior form of relaxation, and you will find the ability to relax helpful when the time comes for prenatal tests, having your baby, and coping with a cesarean recovery and a new baby at the same time. If you are interested in yoga, I recommend *Yoga for New Parents* by Ferris Urbanowski.

RELAXATION BREATHING TECHNIQUES

Every prepared childbirth program worthy of its name readies couples for labor and delivery by means of relaxation breathing techniques. There are different techniques with various names (Lamaze, Kitzinger, Bing, etc.), but the purpose of each one is to train the mind through control and concentration to alleviate the discomforts of labor. Why then do cesarean mothers need these skills?

Braxton-Hicks Contractions. During pregnancy the cesarean mother experiences these testing contractions, which ready the uterus for labor. Remember, your uterus doesn't know it won't have to be prepared for labor. (For more information about Braxton-Hicks contractions, see Chapter 6, Signs of Labor and What to Do.)

Pelvic Examinations. Internal examinations do not usually hurt, but they can be embarrassing, uncomfortable, or tension-producing. Relaxation breathing techniques will be helpful whenever you have to have an internal examination.

Delivery. During delivery it is still possible to feel minor sensation even with a spinal or epidural anesthetic. These sensations may feel like pressure, pulling, or tugging. (For

more information, see Chapter 8, Birthday!) These sensations
do not mean that the anesthesia has failed to work, but you
will want to know how to relax to reduce discomfort.

*Postpartum Contractions.*Within a very short time after the
baby has been born, your uterus will start to contract to its
normal nonpregnant size. These postpartum uterine contractions are similar to labor contractions. Relaxation breathing
will help you to cope.

Postpartum Discomfort. Uncomfortable feelings after
delivery range from mild to acute. Formerly effortless movements such as turning, sitting, walking, sneezing, and coughing,
may be painful for a few days. Controlled, relaxed breathing
will help you to cope more comfortably and effectively.

Tests of Fetal Maturity and Well-Being. These tests are being
used more frequently today and may be stress-producing
stituations. Relaxation breathing will be helpful if your doctor
orders an amniocentesis or stress test. (See Chapter 5, Tests
to Determine Fetal Maturity and Well-Being.)

Most Westerners think of these techniques as a sort of
Oriental mumbo-jumbo. There is no mumbo-jumbo involved,
no arcane mysticism. If need be, a nurse can teach you some
of the more salient points of relaxation breathing techniques
in just a few minutes. But why wait until you are experiencing
extreme anxiety or discomfort before availing yourself of
these methods? It is a skill that can be acquired in just a few
minutes (though practice is helpful), and it is one that will
stand you in good stead for the rest of your life. Even when
your childbearing years are over, there will still be times when
you become tense. Within the context of pregnancy and childbirth, relaxation breathing techniques are a tool, a valuable
resource on which to draw to "stay on top" of tension or
discomfort.

Controlled Relaxation Breathing. The easiest technique is
called Controlled Breathing. It can be done at any time, anywhere, and does not require special equipment or preparation.
Take a deep breath in and then let out all the air. (This

breath is called a welcoming breath). It will provide you with additional oxygen. Then breathe in slowly through your nose to the count of one, two, three. On the count of three, begin to let the air out through pursed lips, again to the count of one, two, three. Do this several times (as necessary). To end the exercise, take another deep breath (a relaxation or parting breath) in, and let it out. You might want to time yourself, or have a partner time you. Use 30, 60, and 90 seconds as intervals of time in which to practice.

Dissociative Breathing and Touch Relaxation. When you become tense emotionally, the muscles in your body become tense, too. Conversely, if part of your body becomes tense, or is subjected to an unwelcome pain stimulus, your mind will tense up. You will want to know how to control your mind to relax your body. In other words, you will want to block out the pain stimuli so that they are unable to maintain control over your thought processes.

To practice dissociative breathing techniques and touch relaxation, it is better to have a partner who can keep a close check on you and help you be aware of parts of your body that are still tense.

Lie on your side, and place pillows under your head and between your knees (which should be flexed) on a bed, mat, or floor with several layers of blanket under you. It is better to practice on your left side to keep the full weight of the baby off the vena cava. [See page 24.] The object of this practice is to achieve a deep sense of relaxation for both your muscles and your mind.

Determine if you feel more comfortable with your eyes open or closed by practicing both ways. If your eyes are open, concentrate on a shape. Don't glare at the shape—that will only increase the tension. Simply use it for a focal area. (An excellent focal area is the face of your mate or coach. Posters, paintings, and mobiles also make good focal areas.)

Take a deep welcoming breath in and let it out. Then, as you breathe in slowly through your nose and out through

pursed lips, imagine that your body is melting, that it has
become as limp as a rag doll or a plate of overcooked spa-
ghetti. When you begin to practice, it may be necessary to give
messages to all the muscles to relax. Start at your toes, tell
them to relax. Work your way up so that every part of your
body becomes soft and relaxed. Continue to breathe in slowly
through your nose, then let the breath out through your
mouth (which will probably be slack if you are comfortable
and relaxing well). While you are doing this controlled, gentle
breathing, your coach should be able to lift any part of you
and feel its entire and total weight in his/her hands. You offer
no resistance. You cannot help to pick up or put down the
arm or leg your coach is supporting. When the time interval
(clocked by the coach) is over, s/he will release your arm or
leg. Take a deep parting breath in and let it out. Practice your
breathing exercises several times a day. When the session is
over, remember that you should *not* go suddenly from a
position flat on the floor to a full sit or stand. If you do, you
may become dizzy. As Sheila Kitzinger, a noted British childbirth educator, advises, whenever you get up after lying down,
pretend that you are Cleopatra rising slowly and elegantly
from her barge. Cleopatra would not have jumped up like a
rabbit. You shouldn't either. Always, always turn on your
side, rest there until you want to stand, and use your hands to
help lift your body. If you try to accomplish a straight sit-up
when getting out of bed or finishing your relaxation breathing
practice session, you'll find the strain on your abdominal
muscles great.

To help determine what you look like when you are relaxed, your coach should observe you while you are sound
asleep. If your coach is your mate, he will know which parts of
your body are most likely to be more tense than others. Some
people squint their eyes, others tighten the muscles in their
forehead or back, some grit their teeth or clench their jaws or
fist. After a few practice sessions, your coach should be able
to pinch you (hard!) on any part of your body. If you have

become well versed in dissociative breathing techniques, you will be aware of the pressure, but not the pain.

If your background includes yoga, meditation, or any similar discipline, relaxation will be almost second nature to you. The important thing is to devise a means of transcending the physical plane in a manner that works well for you. You may want to focus on a shape, silently chant a word or phrase, or envision a lovely scene.

Proficiency in relaxation and controlled breathing techniques is every bit as helpful to the cesarean mother as it is to any other expectant mother. If you spend only five or ten minutes a day practicing (with an occasional day off as a sort of positive stroke to the ego) you will have sufficient time to learn how to control your mind and body in order to conquer discomfort and tension.

TELLING THE CHILDREN

Most children assume that babies come out of the mother's tummy—after all, that's where they grow. Thus, explaining the cesarean delivery to a child can sometimes be easier than explaining a vaginal delivery. However, you should explain to children that there are two ways of having a baby. How much you tell them, and when, will depend on your children's ages and how comfortable you feel with the subject.

Pregnancy is a good time to introduce the subject of how babies are made. Little children will be fascinated to feel the baby kick sometimes. It makes the new baby seem more real to them and in the long run will probably help to reduce the amount of sibling jealousy.

It is also important to explain to children that you will need to spend a few days in the hospital when the baby is born. It's rather an unpleasant surprise for children not to know that mummy will be leaving for a few days and then have her return home with an "intruder" in her arms.

Mothers are usually more concerned about hospitalization

than children. Just as long as the children are happy with the person who takes care of them and have special activities planned, mother's absence will probably have little negative effect. Crying and being sad that mother has to go away for a few days is normal. Little children's sense of time is not well developed and they probably won't be as aware of how long she is gone as the mother is. In fact, many a mother has returned home to find her older children paying more attention to the television or a toy than to her! All the time she thought they'd be pining away, they've been having a good time doing things with Grandma or Auntie their parents would never let them do!

CHAPTER 4 EMOTIONAL STRESS:
THE FEAR FACTOR

These comments were made by parents who had no preparation to help them cope with an emergency cesarean delivery. All echo the need for education and support.

"I'm just not ready to be a mother."

"The responsibilities of fatherhood are overwhelming. Why are we having a baby now?"

"I shouldn't have been in such a hurry to have a baby. I had a career I really liked."

"Maybe we should have waited longer . . . paid off the house . . . traveled more . . . become more secure financially."

"Bill and I really wanted this baby. We planned to have it. It wasn't an accident. We waited until we thought we were ready. Now I don't know. Some days I feel trapped. I'm scared. How are we going to be able to cope?"

"I'm afraid my baby will be deformed or retarded."

"I'm afraid the strain of having another baby will destroy our relationship. It's so fragile now. Herb wasn't much help after the first one. How's he going to react this time?"

These feelings may be voiced by *any* parent and are probably no more or less acute in cesarean pregnancies. But there can be an additional stress with a cesarean pregnancy. Here are some reactions from cesarean parents-to-be:

"I'm afraid to have another section. The first one was awful. I was in labor for what seemed like years before I had the section. It hurt so much afterwards, too. It took me six months before I felt like a real human being again. I didn't even know that the baby had been born until the next day.

41

When I woke up, I thought I was still in labor. I'm so afraid
to go through that again. But now it's too late. For me it's the
only way I can have a baby."

"I'm happy to be pregnant again. It took so long to conceive the first baby. Then I had two miscarriages before this
pregnancy. I really do want this baby. But I hate the thought
of getting anesthesia and being all cut up again."

"I thought I was going to die. They kept giving me something to bring on contractions and then they'd zonk me out
with something else. I was so lonely and confused by that
time. When they said they were going to do a cesarean, I welcomed the announcement. I think what bothered me more
than anything was that there were a bunch of interns around
my bed. They kept talking about me as though I was a
cadaver. They said things to each other like, 'Her pulse is
failing.' and 'I can't get the baby's heartbeat.' There were a
lot of other women in that big room and they were all moan-
ing, 'Help me, help me, please. Won't somebody help me, I'm
dying.' This was my first baby so I assumed they knew more
than I did. If they were dying, I figured I might be, too. And
when the interns said they couldn't get the baby's heartbeat,
it meant my baby was dead. The final, ultimate insult was to
hear one of them say, 'The full moon sure brought out a
bunch of weirdos.' So there I was, a dying weirdo with a dead
baby. My son was born healthy, but it wasn't thanks to the
tender, loving care I got."

"I know I should feel grateful. I would have died, and the
baby, too, if I had lived fifty or a hundred years ago. But the
section was so unplanned. We didn't want to be pulled away
from each other when the going got tough. The doctor made
Jerry leave, and I wanted him to stay. He left, but not will-
ingly. At the hospital where I'm going fathers are not allowed
to be with their wives at all for a section. It's so sad really.
This is our last baby. We wanted to share the first one's birth,
and now we won't even be able to be together for this one.
I wish there was something we could do."

"My mother had two cesareans. She said she almost died

each time. She was so afraid she'd get pregnant again that she wouldn't let my father touch her. But that was many years ago. More than anything in the world, I wanted to avoid having a section. I was floored when the doctor said the baby was breech and that I might have to have a cesarean. It wasn't as bad as I thought it would be, but it wasn't very nice. The doctor tried to give me a spinal and it didn't work so I got put out. I hated it. I couldn't believe how much pain there was afterwards. I'm afraid. I don't want to have to go through the pain again. Other women say it isn't so awful to have a cesarean . . . but I don't know . . . it sure hurt like hell."

"Doctors charge an extra fee for doing a section. It's such a rip-off. It probably takes them less time, especially with a repeat 'cause they can schedule when they have to come in. It takes only an hour. Sometimes they have to spend hours and hours waiting in the hospital while a woman's in labor. They shouldn't charge extra for doing a cesarean—they should charge less. Cesarean parents have to pay extra for everything. It's a form of discrimination, and I don't like it. Besides, we can't afford to have a baby. I'm really worried about all those bills. I got pregnant and then my husband got laid off so we don't have any insurance. You've gotta be either extra-rich or extra-poor in order to get medical care. If you're in the middle like us, you pay through the nose."

"I had my appendix out a few years ago. They almost burst right before Thanksgiving dinner. I wasn't scared then. I was in too much pain, and it was the first time anyone had paid me that much attention. I was just glad to get it over with. Two years ago I had an emergency c-sec. I was scared to death. Appendix are one thing, but a baby, why, that's something else. I was afraid I would die. I was afraid the doctor would cut the baby by accident. I was afraid my guts would spill out onto the floor the first time I got out of bed. I was afraid to hold the baby. I was afraid I wouldn't be a good mother. I was afraid to take the baby home. I felt lousy. It was so hard, taking care of a baby and getting over the opera-

tion. When I had my appendix out, I could go home and rest and recuperate. It was the same kind of thing—the operation, that is. I mean it's done almost the same way. But my appendix weren't handed to me wrapped in a blanket for feedings at 2 a.m."

"What was the best part? Geeze, there wasn't any good part. It was all pretty bad, I mean, aside from having a beautiful baby and all. You know, I think the doctor really genuinely thinks he did a good job. I mean, he did spend a lot of time with me when I went to his office. But he never really answered my questions. He just sort of said, 'Well, it's okay. Just leave everything to me.' When I was in the hospital, the nurses made me feel like I was bothering them when I called for help. I tried not to think about myself too much, and concentrated on the baby. But it hurt a lot. I didn't want my husband to think I wasn't happy to have the baby. I was. But I don't want to go through that again. Not alone, not without someone to understand how I felt, how much help I needed. I hate being dependent on anyone. But I really had to lean on everyone, the nurses, my husband, and my mother who came to help after the baby was born."

"None of my friends had sections. They made me feel like a weirdo for not being able to do it 'their' way, the 'right' way. After a while, I didn't even want to see them again. They were so condescending. They did everything within a week after the baby was born. I was still in the hospital. Then when I got home I felt like a zombie. Oh, they complained about their long labors and their episiotomies and their hemorrhoids. But I had a long, hard labor, too, and a huge stomach cut and hemorrhoids."

"It's too bad there isn't any information for cesareans. It would have made things a lot easier on us if we could have found out about it before it happened."

"I didn't know what to expect, and when it was all over, I didn't know what had happened, only that it did happen. I wish I knew what happened, and why, and how my baby was *born. I felt like we were functioning in a vacuum. I get scared when I don't know what to expect. It's a lot better—and easier to deal with—if you know what's going to happen, and how it's going to feel. I want the next baby to be born while I'm awake. It's kind of like the difference between giving birth under a bushel basket, and having a baby out in the open."*

"My mother told me never to get pregnant again after I had my first cesarean. When I did, she told me I'd better take out a life insurance policy on myself 'cause I'd never make it off the operating table alive."

"I know this isn't true only of cesarean mothers, but I felt like a pawn in a chess game. I chose to go to a certain doctor because I heard he was real good. But when I got to my first visit, I was told, not asked, that I would see a different one of the three doctors each time. Well, I know I shouldn't say this but . . . I really took an instant disliking to one of them. The other one was okay. My face must have dropped down to the floor each time someone other than 'my' doctor came into the room—the first time especially. I think there's something very important about establishing a good relationship with your doctor. It can be a father-daughter relationship, or a brother/sister thing, or a friend-to-friend kind of thing. I resented the fact that I was paying for the services of one doctor, and had to settle for the other ones. It was my money, and I felt terrible but I was too intimidated to speak up. I tried it once, with the receptionist, but all she said was, 'That's just the way we do things here. It's better for you to see all the doctors. You can't do it your way.' I dropped the subject after that. It was too much trouble to pursue it, and I didn't want to hurt the other doctors' feelings. It was just my rotten luck to get the one I liked least to do the cesarean. I felt disappointed. I think I wouldn't have minded so much if I'd gotten the doctor I liked best."

"The only thing I could find out about cesarean sections was that there wasn't any information. So I asked around. All I heard were scare stories. So I stopped asking."

"Hal and I bought every book on childbirth we could find. I'd come back from the library with so many books I could hardly hold them all. We read every word. Then I had a surprise cesarean. So I went back to those books and looked up the word. You know what? Some of them didn't even mention it! And in others, there was so little as to be almost useless. Usually it didn't even say anything about cesareans, other than that it was an operation. What killed me were the ones that said you could avoid having a section if you minded your p's and q's. Hey, I did that! I was really looking forward to having my first baby. And I was religious about practicing and exercising. I was better about doing my exercises and breathing than anyone else in our class! So I felt like a failure and an ignorant fool. What concerns me is that I want to make the next birth better. I want it to be a good thing, not only for me, but for my baby and husband. He felt so cheated. I don't want it to be the horror show it was before, although mine wasn't as bad as some of the women I've talked to. But I am very much afraid. I know I shouldn't be, but I know that anesthesia can be dangerous. . . . I know that the baby can be born with breathing problems like the Kennedy baby. . . . I know that I could get a terrible infection . . . and I know that I'm being too much of a worry-wart. My head tells me that everythng will be all right. But my heart says, 'Look out, with your luck, anything that could go wrong will.' "

The "fear factor" of a cesarean birth can involve many things including:

1. The responsibilities of parenthood.

2. The loss of income if the mother has been working, coupled with the extra cost of a cesarean delivery, and the financial strain of supporting another child.

3. Fear that the baby will be less than perfect, that she will be damaged or defective.

4. Guilt that negative emotions crop up at a time in one's life when everything is *supposed* to be beautiful and perfect

. . . when the anticipation of a new baby is *supposed* to bring joy, not resentment.

5. The fears of *any* person about to undergo any type of surgery. These fears are accented in the case of cesarean parents, for the family will be simultaneously involved in *both* childbirth *and* surgery.

6. The almost total lack of solid, helpful information. Couples have often had to rely on myths, misinformation, and old wives' tales. The experiences of other cesarean mothers, who may relate tales of horror, however true or false these impressions may be, undermine much of the confidence pregnant cesarean couples have developed on their own.

7. Memory of previous experiences that may have been fraught with pain and/or psychological and physical stress.

8. Condescension by one's peers who may see the cesarean mother as a failure. This attitude, combined with the fact that the mother may already feel inadequate, is sufficient to create numerous problems.

8. Possible lack of rapport between doctor and client as à result of personality conflict, the lack of alternative doctors and/or hospitals (as is the case in areas where the population is not dense enough to give expectant couples a choice), specialization (a different doctor is called in to treat various members of each family, and different medical conditions for each member) or the growing number of team practices that do not take into account the fact that the woman may not wish to be cared for by all members of the group, but prefers one doctor to the others.

10. The lack of prenatal classes and support groups for expectant cesarean parents in many areas of the country.

11. The lack of postpartum help and support for the cesarean mother both in the hospital and after returning home.

Women who deliver vaginally and who have had very negative birth experiences do not relish the thought of going through "that" again, and the prospect of an elective or repeat cesarean may carry with it the same impact as knowing almost

Recipe

Take: two parents-to-be who may experience a temporary panic as they contemplate the responsibilities of parenthood and their unpreparedness for taking care of a newborn

Add: a dash of fear that the baby may be born less than perfect

Fold in: the parents' guilt that they are having negative thoughts in the first place

Combine: the ordinary trepidations of anyone about to have surgery

Take away: books, films, and slides concerning this alternative birthing method (because there haven't been any)

Remove: classes in prepared childbirth designed to meet the special needs of these parents (Because no one thought they were needed)

Beat in: two lumps of confusion on behalf of maternity personnel who are not quite certain about their roles in caring for a patient who is both postpartum and postsurgical

Throw in: anxiety, tension, myths and misinformation—and the often harrowing experiences of others

Separate: parents just when they need each other's love and support most

Optional: one or more previous cesarean deliveries

Wheel: your mixture into an operating room and keep there for about one hour, or until done

Yield: one cesarean section, one hopefully healthy baby, and two traumatized parents

a full year in advance that you have an appointment with a particularly sadistic dentist. The anticipation of childbirth-cum-surgery or surgery-cum-childbirth as the case may be is the major "fear factor" in cesarean pregnancies *unless* cesarean parents are given the skills needed to help themselves achieve better birthing experiences.

How many women sail through a cesarean delivery with nary a negative thought and without a moment's pain? Surely, there are some who do not find the experience the least bit difficult, trying, or disconcerting. Others may be so happy to have a baby after years of infertility that the result more than justifies the means: a healthy baby after years of waiting. However, women who find the experience easy and completely without discomfort or tension are probably in the minority.

The keys to alleviating the additional psychological stress of a cesarean delivery are education and empathy. That tired old phrase, "We have nothing to fear but fear itself" has special meaning for cesarean couples. Knowing what to expect and how to cope is the best preparation and the only defense against fear.

Enlightenment follows education. As information about cesarean childbirth becomes more widely available, traditional attitudes will change. Many cesarean parents are developing a new raised consciousness, which will extend from these parents to doctors, nurses, hospital administrators, childbirth educators, friends, family, and everyone with whom cesarean parents come into contact. Where the cesarean mother may have been neither "fish nor fowl" previously (she was not just a postsurgical patient, nor was she *only* a regular postpartum maternity patient) and could not therefore be neatly categorized as "ordinary," she will now benefit from a new status that takes into account her very special physical and emotional needs.

Empathy is needed from everyone who comes into contact with cesarean parents, be it on a friendship or professional basis. Friends can learn to respect the cesarean mother, rather than look down on her. Families need no longer feel "sorry" for her. Childbirth educators will no longer see these couples as "oddities" or "failures" who didn't follow their advice, instruction, and rules. Cesarean parents do not want to be smothered in sympathy or coldly rejected—but they *do* need empathy, education, support, encouragement, and a new understanding of their special needs.

Anyone who has ever had major surgery can remember the difficulties involved. Anyone who has ever had a baby knows what child care entails. We should ask, "What must it feel like to have a baby *and* an operation?" "Should we expect cesarean women to automatically, magically transform themselves into 'good' and caring mothers at a time when their own physical limitations make them potentially (and very understandably) egocentric?" Any parent who has had a baby by cesarean knows the answers. As one nurse said, "I thought cesarean mothers were a big pain in the neck. They were always calling the station for help. Then I got pregnant and had to have a c-section. Boy, did my attitude change in a hurry!"

It is not necessary for a childbirth instructor to have a cesarean to teach cesarean couples—but it helps. Male doctors, however well-intentioned, cannot know how their clients feel—but they *can* empathize. Regarding their patients as pregnant uteri that must be incised may help doctors in their job of objectively making decisions—but it does not encourage their understanding of their clients as people. The nurse or doctor who has never had a baby, or who had a vaginal delivery, or who delivered so many years ago that there were few differences between how mothers were treated regardless of the method of delivery can still be a tremendous help to the cesarean family.

Health care professionals can begin to reassess their attitudes. They could start by imagining how they would feel if a doctor or nurse walked into their rooms and said (as some doctors and nurses are now saying), "Stop blubbering. Stop bemoaning your fate. You had a baby. It's healthy. Why are you so upset? It's nothing. You'll get over it." The nurse who breezes into the room of a newly delivered cesarean mother, leaves the baby's crib ten feet away from the mother's bed, and then zips out almost as quickly as she came in might stop a minute to picture how she would feel if she were the mother in that bed. Most nurses are *not* callous or unconcerned. The problem has often been that some nurses simply have never given much thought to the plight of the cesarean mother who is (initially) quite physically handicapped, who may feel help-less, alone, frightened, or uncomfortable, and who is com-pletely unable to get out of bed without assistance—much less get the baby back into bed with her. Cesarean fathers who find themselves short on understanding might also try to put them-selves in their wives' situation. How would they feel being uncomfortable physically and almost totally dependent on others for help?

In-service training programs are now being offered in a number of hospitals to increase the level of understanding with regard to present systems of care for cesarean families. News-papers and magazines are catching on to the fact that articles about "cesarean sections" are timely and of interest to readers. Childbirth education associations are to be credited with im-proving the care and handling of vaginal deliveries. Now, fortunately, many of them are devoting some effort to taking the cesarean "section" out of the dark ages. Slowly but surely people are beginning to see the cesarean delivery in a new light.

"I just never thought about it that way" is a remark fre-quently made by health care professionals, childbirth educa-tors, editors, and noncesarean parents. Because the majority of cesarean deliveries performed today are *technically* perfect, the very false assumption has been that there is no need to concern oneself with the *emotional* well-being of cesarean couples. Unless cesarean couples speak up and speak out, it is possible for hundreds of poor quality (from the psychological aspect) cesarean deliveries to take place without anyone in the hospital giving the procedure, or the people who have experi-enced it, more than passing thought. The doctor may admire the precision of the incision, the neatness of the scar. The anesthesiologist may wonder at the ease with which the anesthesia was administered. Nurses may congratulate themselves on their efficiency. And the parents may be totally drained by the experience. They take their babies home from the hospital thinking that they are glad to be out of there, and wondering why they don't feel more grateful for such expert care.

It is difficult, if not impossible, for many people to express their concerns. If previous cesarean deliveries were harrowing, and left bitter impressions, the results can sometimes be measured by the degree of withdrawal, fright, hostility or displaced anger experienced. Often, cesarean parents simply "grin and bear it," "keep a stiff upper lip," and adhere to all the other clichés about keeping one's problems to oneself. If cesarean parents do not talk about how they feel, no one is going to know how to help them. Organizations of cesarean parents, for cesarean parents, are being formed in many areas throughout the country. They are excellent sources of information and support. Together cesarean parents will be able to talk about their experiences with others who can truly understand. Together they will be able to work through and finalize the experience, and move on to more positive attitudes. Together they will share tips on how to cope with situations as diverse as anesthesia and simultaneous care of both a dependent toddler and a new baby in the first few weeks at home. Together they can achieve better quality health care for themselves and for future cesarean parents as well.

Doctors, hospital administrators, childbirth educators, and maternity nurses should be approached with determination but not obsession about the goals, complaints, questions, and comments of cesarean parents. They will probably be quite willing to listen to suggestions. If they are doing their jobs well in their own eyes, suggestions for change may meet with initial resistance. Give them time. You may have been thinking about the subject for weeks or months, but your suggestions are *new* to them. Be patient, persistent, and above all, polite.

Empathy cannot grow in a climate of hostility or aggression. But it *will* come with time and understanding. Today's cesarean parents will pave the way for better quality birth experiences for themselves and make the going easier for future cesarean parents.

There may not be enough time to achieve all your goals while you are pregnant. But your efforts will not be in vain, for they *will* help others. Your enthusiasm will be passed on to other cesarean parents, to your children, to family, friends, and health care professionals.

Cesarean mothers do not have to live in fear of the impending delivery. With the sharing of efforts and the cooperation of others, they can look forward to a birthing experience that is positive, joyous, and comfortable. As understanding grows, tension and fear will decrease. There should be *no* stigma associated with having a cesarean delivery. It can and should be regarded as an alternative method of giving birth, an experience to be met with confidence and joy.

AFTER DELIVERY

If the trauma of the birth has left scars on a woman's psyche, they may not fade as quickly as the one on her abdomen, and it may be necessary for her to seek professional counseling. Usually, though, a psychological distance and lapse of time between the mother and her birth experience will help put negative feelings in perspective. Temporary feelings of anger, resentment, failure, frustration, and/or depression are not unusual.

Unfortunately, until fairly recently many cesarean birth experiences have been harrowing and emotionally stressful. It is also true that a few cesarean mothers use their birth experiences as scapegoats for earlier, unrelated problems such as marital troubles or deep-seated chronic depression. A host of unrelated physical ailments such as frigidity, weight gain, or headaches may also be "blamed" on the cesarean delivery.

In the first few months after delivery the lack of sexual desire may cause the mother to think that she has become frigid. It is difficult—if not impossible—to feel amorous when one has been deprived of a full night's sleep for weeks and the house has fallen into rack and ruin because the baby requires so much time. How *do* new parents find the time to make love even if they want to? It can be arranged, but not always easily. (For a further discussion, see "The Fourth Trimester".) If a woman gains weight, it is not because she had a cesarean, but because she is eating too much. Headaches as the result of anesthesia sometimes do occur—but if they do, they will happen within a few days of delivery, not months later.

The cesarean mother may harbor resentment against the baby for being too big or in the wrong position to have been delivered vaginally or for taking up so much of her time after birth; against the doctor for not letting her know what was happening, for allowing her to be in labor so long before making the decision to do a cesarean, or for not allowing her to labor longer to see if she could deliver vaginally; against the nurses for interfering too much or not enough; against the baby's father for making her pregnant in the first place, or for not coaching and supporting her well enough. The list is endless, and not without contradictions.

The new cesarean mother may be angry with herself for accepting or rejecting medication; she may hate her body for being too small, too uncooperative to allow her to have her baby vaginally. She may well think she did something wrong. Birth is supposed to be a normal, natural event. And she could not do it "right." No matter what the indications for her cesarean, no matter what she did or did not do, the fact remains that for the remainder of her life she may have unresolved questions and doubts. "If only I knew then what I know now, I could have avoided a cesarean." "If only I hadn't given up so soon, I might have avoided a cesarean." "If only I had practiced my exercises more." "If I could just do it again, things would be different." "If only. . . ."

Frustration may come as the result of listening to friends who have had beautiful, shared vaginal deliveries. They can talk so glowingly of their babies' births . . . and the cesarean mother may not even be able to remember hers, much less have been able to share it with the baby's father. Her sense of control, her sense of accomplishment have been taken from her.

Depression immediately after childbirth is a commonly accepted medical condition. No one can as yet accurately predict who will get it, why it happens, and what can be done to prevent it. The new cesarean mother may feel like a fool for crying in front of the nurse when she brings in the umpteenth bowl of jello—and the mother is so hungry she could eat a six-course dinner for two. Her husband may be bewildered by her actions when she comes home from the hospital. He cannot understand why she's crying because the baby that they (especially she) wanted and waited for is crying. She may reach the point where she is unable to cope unless she vents her feelings.

No one told the new mother—nor would she have believed—that being a mother can be complicated, time consuming, and almost devoid of creativity and adult companionship. Women pregnant for the first time are notorious for romanticizing what it will be like when the baby comes. They imagine themselves ideal mothers with ideal babies. The reality is that the mother may be crying because she is just as tired, hungry, and in need of love as her baby. The baby's needs have priority. The mother's needs for gratification must be delayed. There are rewards to being a mother—but they may not be apparent for weeks. In the meantime, during the day, the only companionship the mother may have is the television and her baby.

Unless the depression is major and long lasting (in which case the mother will want to see a therapist), it is small consolation to know that she is not alone in her feelings. The best thing she can do is to find other women who are in the same postcesarean, postpartum, new-baby predicament. A local parents' support group or an instructor of prenatal classes should be able to put the mother in touch with other new parents. *Any* new mother (regardless of the method of delivery) is likely to be in the same situation.

Crying is a good release. One should not feel guilty for being resentful, angry, frustrated, or depressed—it will only compound the problem. No one is ever admonished for feeling happy, generous, kind, or virtuous—but most of us feel something is intrinsically wrong if we let negative feelings surface. There is something wrong if sad and angry is the only feeling experienced all the time. If you are feeling down because you are exhausted and have been through an upheaval that is both physically and emotionally traumatic (the cesarean delivery and a baby to care for), you have a right to be on edge, uptight, or blue.

Postpartum depression may be a commonly accepted medical condition—but there is nothing "routine" about it. It is devastating. Its incidence is so great that it should be considered a possibility whenever depressed feelings are very intense or persistent.

It is not wrong to experience *temporary* negative feelings after the baby is born. You may have felt any of these emotions even if your baby had been delivered vaginally, and all your dreams of the "perfect" birth came true. However, there may be a greater sense of failure with a cesarean birth. You didn't fail, but you may think you did. This sense of incompetence may be greater among women whose first cesareans were unplanned. If you are physically exhausted, exhaustion may intensify your feelings of being unable to cope. You may also be jealous of women who have had vaginal births. (It is sometimes hard to appreciate, but some women actually envy cesarean mothers because they don't have to go through labor again!) But it does not help to dwell on depression and to be incapacitated by it.

Eventually it should be possible for you to have more

positive feelings about your birth experience. These good
feelings may come when time has elapsed since the baby's
birth. If you have given birth during the winter months the
depression may be greater. As spring comes, you may begin
to feel lighter and more agreeable. This will also happen when
your baby begins to develop a more manageable routine.
Babies are demanding little creatures. The first time your baby
smiles at you may just coincide with the end of much of your
depression. At last the baby seems to be giving, rather than
taking. It is good to express one's negative feelings—but it
is not constructive to dwell on them entirely. If you hear
yourself sounding like a broken record, it's time to change the
tune. You may not be able to accomplish it singlehandedly.
You will need the help of your husband, family and close
friends. Feedback and support from other cesarean parents
and concerned professionals can be very beneficial, too. The
end product of really working through one's sadness or grief
should be a greater ability to accept what happened—even if
you still have some negative feelings about it. You may wish to
channel your negative feelings into something constructive
such as writing letters or articles, helping other cesarean
parents, and working for improvements so that parents may
benefit from your experiences.

A cesarean birth is not always easy—but, in the words of
one mother, "It doesn't have to be so hard. If you know what
might happen, you can deal with anything."

CHAPTER 5 TESTS TO DETERMINE FETAL MATURITY AND WELL-BEING

*T*HE 1970's brought sophisticated new tests and machines to the field of obstetrics. While these tests may be employed for any pregnancy, they are of outstanding value in repeat and elective cesarean deliveries.

Until the introduction of these tests, repeat and elective cesarean births were routinely scheduled to take place about ten days to two weeks before the estimated date of delivery. It takes approximately forty weeks of gestation for the human baby to fully develop and mature. The problem is that babies do not read the books on pregnancy that tell them how long it requires. Some babies take longer than others to ready their systems for life outside the uterus. Prior to the introduction of these new tests, the obstetrician, in scheduling a cesarean delivery, had to rely on time-honored, but less than infallible considerations such as the mother's estimated date of conception (a date that is likely to be in error), when the mother first felt the baby move (quickening), the height of the fundus (top of the uterus), and signs within the mother's body, such as dilation of the cervix (neck of the uterus), which would indicate that labor was near.

The doctor took these factors into consideration, along with the woman's medical history, and hoped that s/he had scheduled an optimal time for both mother and baby and that the baby would be born healthy, full-term, and really able to function independently outside the mother's body. These computations and considerations amounted, in essence, to erudite guesswork. There was no way to gauge surely and accurately what stage of gestation the fetus had reached, nor how well she was progressing in utero. This problem resulted in the traditionally higher incidence of respiratory distress syndrome among cesarean-delivered babies.

Respiratory Distress Syndrome (RDS)—a newer and more accurate name for hyaline membrane disease—is a condition wherein the air sacs (alveoli) of the lungs are unable to stay open as they should, and collapse after each breath the baby takes. The infant has to work strenuously with each new breath, and soon develops numerous physiological and metabolic problems.

Because the incidence of RDS has been higher among cesarean-delivered babies, it became customary to place all cesarean babies in the special care nursery for an observation period of approximately 12 to 24 hours, regardless of birth weight, Apgar score, or general condition. (It is a wise precaution, but one that is by no means always necessary.) In special care nurseries, the baby is placed in an isolette (incubator) and the staff watches for possible signs of distress. Special equipment is available should any problems arise.

Tests to determine fetal maturity and well-being are now reducing the risk of RDS and of scheduling a cesarean delivery before the baby is prepared to function independently. The cesarean mother-to-be may have any one or a combination of these tests. She probably will not have all of them. The major consideration is to schedule the birth at a time when the baby is ready. A healthy, full-term infant is the prime concern of both the parents and obstetrician.

Ultrasound or Sonargram. Until fairly recently, X ray was the only way to determine the size of the fetus and the mother's pelvic outlet. Precautions are taken to diminish the danger of radiation to the baby, but the risk of contamination is one doctors prefer to avoid if possible. Should your doctor order X rays for you, bear in mind that a minimum amount of radiation will be used, and that the danger of X ray is not as great as it once was. Now it is used sparingly, and the days when whole series of many X rays were considered necessary are over.

Today some hospitals and clinics have a machine called an Ultrasound or Sonargram. Instead of X ray, the machine uses ultrahigh frequency sound waves. This machine—the names ultrasound and sonargram are interchangeable—takes a "picture" of the fetus and placenta. The sonargram can determine the size of the fetus relative to gestational age, its position, the placement of the placenta, and/or multiple births. The cost of the machine (about $25,000) and its relative newness means that not all hospitals have it as yet.

Each ultrasound series is expensive (approximately $50 to $100 or more) but it is painless and harmless to both mother and baby. The only preparation is that the mother should have a full bladder. A full bladder will show up clearly on the picture and can be used as a landmark for interpretation, and during the later stages of pregnancy, a full bladder is not a difficult feat to accomplish. In fact, most pregnant women find that keeping the bladder empty is far harder.

The procedure takes just minutes to complete. The abdomen is covered with an oily substance (baby oil, olive oil, lanolin, or another lotion) to facilitate running the device, which resembles a microphone, back and forth over the abdomen. It is a good idea to wear clothing that will not be ruined should some oil remain on the abdomen after the test is completed.

Sonargram pictures do not look like "real babies" to most of us. It is not a photographic image, but a graph composed of a series of dots. Polaroid pictures of the test results are sometimes offered to the parents. Even though you may not be able to interpret them, these pictures are nice keepsakes to have.

L/S Ratio. The unborn baby is surrounded by amniotic

fluid, which among other things, washes into and out of the
fetal lungs. It also serves as a protective cushion should the
mother experience a blow to her abodmen. As recently as ten
to fifteen years ago, the information its properties contained
was all but unknown. Now laboratory tests of the amniotic
fluid can help to determine such conditions as Rh-sensitized
pregnancies, genetic makeup, and fetal lung maturity. The test
to determine fetal lung maturity, called an "l/s ratio," is the
one which has the most relevance for cesarean parents. Once
the uterus is opened, the doctor cannot say, "Hmm, this baby
is having difficulty breathing, I think I'll put her back in for
a while." The l/s ratio is a new sophisticated means to make
certain that the baby is born at a time when her lungs are
mature.

   Among the substances found in the amniotic fluid are
lecithin and sphingomyelin. It is now possible to predict
quite accurately how mature the fetal lungs are by comparing
the amount of lecithin to the amount of sphingomyelin.
Until about the thirty-fifth week of gestation, the quantities
of these two substances are approximately equal. After the
thirty-fifth week, the proportion of lecithin becomes increasingly greater. Only when the baby's lungs are mature enough
to function independently will the proportion of lecithin
increase. When there is at least twice as much lecithin, it is
safe to schedule the cesarean. It is not important to memorize
the words lecithin and sphingomyelin, but rather to know
what a valuable resource the l/s ratio is for scheduling elective
and repeat cesarean deliveries at a time when the baby's lungs
are mature, and thus reduce the possibility of respiratory
distress syndrome.

   To take a small sample of the amniotic fluid, the obstetrician will do an *amniocentesis* (pronounced "am-nee-oh-sen-
tee-sis"). Another name for the procedure is "amniotic tap,"
or simply a "tap." When a small quantity of amniotic fluid has
been obtained, it will be sent to a laboratory for analysis.

   Don't let the words lecithin, sphingomyelin, and amniocentesis frighten or intimidate you. They are hard to pronounce initially, and are not household words. It is perfectly acceptable and accurate to say "l/s ratio" and "amniotic tap." "Taps" are sometimes performed right in the doctor's office, or in the hospital on an outpatient basis. The doctor may charge an extra fee for this service, and if you go to the hospital to have the test, there will be a charge for use of the facilities (sometimes an emergency examining room is used, or sometimes a regular labor room or clinic examining room).

Probably no other test "scares" expectant parents more than an amniocentesis. At most, a tap is mildly uncomfortable. Once the doctor is ready to begin, it takes just a few minutes to complete. The mother will be given a hospital gown to wear. Before the test starts, make yourself as comfortable and relaxed as possible. Often having a pillow under one's shoulder and another under one's knees is most comfortable. To alleviate emotional tension or physical discomfort, slow, controlled relaxation breathing is advised.

If you're feeling apprehensive about having an l/s ratio done, ask if you can bring your mate or a friend or relative with you for reassurance and support. S/he will be able to help you do some controlled relaxation breathing, and because you will have had nothing to eat or drink for eight hours prior to the test, having someone drive you to and from the doctor's office or hospital is a good safeguard should you feel faint or dizzy from not eating.

The doctor begins by covering your abdomen with a colorful antiseptic solution which may feel cool to you at first. Your doctor may or may not inject a local anesthetic in the abdominal area. Some doctors do not give an injection on the grounds that the discomfort of this local anesthetic is as great as the tap itself. Then, the doctor will take a cannula (a hollow needle) and insert it into your abdomen. You may feel a slight prickling sensation, similar to the feeling of having a blood sample drawn. Because the doctor does not want to encounter either the baby or the placenta, s/he may have to insert the needle several times to get it just right. Care is taken to ascertain that puncture of the placenta does not take place. If you have had an ultrasound test, your doctor will know the location of the placenta. Where the baby is located can also be determined by palpating the abdomen. The doctor will feel your uterus to see what position the baby is in. Some parents worry that the baby will be "jabbed" or "poked" by the cannula. If by chance the baby does get in the way, rest assured that he or she will move! Another parental concern is over the amount of amniotic fluid drawn. The amount of fluid extracted is very small, less than an ounce, and the loss of this tiny quantity will not damage or hurt the baby in any way.

When the amniotic fluid sample has been drawn, a fetal monitor is sometimes used. For the woman who has never before heard her baby's heartbeat, here is an added bonus. Fetal monitors have a volume control in addition to their graphing abilities which can be turned up so that the mother, too, can hear her baby's heart. It is often surprising to hear the fetal heartbeat, for it is about twice the normal adult rate and sounds like a galloping horse. Variations of 120 to 160 beats per minute are average.

If you are put on a fetal monitor, a belt will be placed around your abdomen and you and your baby will be observed for a short time—15 to 30 minutes is average. This period of observation is a precautionary measure. There is a very slight risk of placental puncture. Should this occur, or should the fetal monitor show ominous signs of fetal distress for any reason, the mother will have to remain in the hospital for an immediate cesarean delivery. To be on the safe side, obstetricians usually recommend that all women about to have an amniocentesis abstain from eating and drinking for eight hours prior to the test. Then, if delivery must take place, there will be a lesser risk of complication from the anesthesia. In some hospitals, the mother will be offered something to eat and drink after the test is completed and the observation period is over.

The longest part of the test is the laboratory analysis. At least four hours is required for analysis. Laboratories have different methods of analyzing and evaluating the l/s ratio. In some labs, readings do not exceed 6:1 (six being the greatest amount of lecithin possible according to their methods). Where other methods and rating systems are used, readings can be as high as 8:1, 10:1, and occasionally even 14:1. No matter what methods are used, a reading of 2:1 or higher usually indicates that it is probably quite safe to schedule the baby's birth within a few days.

If a reading of less than 2:1 is taken (for example: 1.5:1), or if the result is very close to 2:1 (such as 2.1:1), and there are no other circumstances which would make waiting longer a potential problem, the physician may ask for a second amniotic tap within a week or so. The amount of lecithin given off by the fetus's lungs can change dramatically within a week's time. The first reading may have been 1.8:1, and a week later, be up to 6:1. The longer the fetus remains in the mother's uterus (in most circumstances), the greater are the chances of the infant's being able to function well on its own.

The results of the l/s ratio will be eagerly awaited by the parents-to-be. If the outcome of the test is a reading of 2:1 or higher, the baby will probably be scheduled for delivery within a day or two. Although the couple has had months and months to prepare for the birth, the very fact that they know when their baby will be born can cause a good case of jitters. It is not uncommon to feel unprepared, even after all the preparations and waiting. Conversely, the results may indicate that the baby prefers to stay right where she is for at least another week. If a low ratio is determined, the pregnant couple (especially the mother) may feel very let down. She may begin to think that her baby will never get born, that she has been pregnant forever, and that the sooner the baby is safely delivered, the happier she will be.

There are two things to remember about an l/s reading. (1) It will *not* tell the sex or chromosomal makeup of the baby. When there is a question about genetics, an amniotic tap is done during the *second* trimester. And (2), if you go into labor spontaneously within a short time after a low l/s ratio reading is determined, it is reassuring to note that the same hormones which stimulate labor may also trigger the baby's respiratory system, and thus diminish the risk of RDS.

Estriol Counts. Estriol is a hormone given off by the fetus which passes through the placenta and into the mother's kidneys. For an estriol count, the mother collects all her urinary output in one container for a period of 24 hours. The urine is then analyzed to determine the level of estriol present. The estriol level will show how well the placenta is functioning, especially when there is a question regarding postmaturity. At least two estriol counts, spaced over a period of a week to ten days, will be taken. Because the quantity of estriol can differ greatly from day to day, at least two counts are necessary.

The test is painless. The only "problem" associated with it is that some women are embarrassed about carrying a plastic container full of urine to the doctor's office, clinic, or lab. Each test costs about $30.00.

Nonstress Test. Nonstress testing is a recent innovation to help determine fetal well-being. The pregnant woman is attached to a Fetal Monitor and a strip (that is, a readout) is run for about 20 minutes. The function of the fetal heart under a normal, nonstressful situation is then noted. The print-out may be used for comparison at a later time (as in stress testing) should it be required.

Stress Test. When there is any doubt about the adequate functioning of the placenta (as may be the case in diabetes, renal disease, toxemia, hypertension, postmaturity, or an absence of fetal movement), a stress test can be given.

For a stress test, the woman is admitted to the hospital and attached to a fetal monitor. An intravenous (i.v.) is started. A sufficient amount of pitocin (a hormone) is given to produce three strong contractions within a 10-minute period.

If the baby's heartbeat remains good during the contractions, it means that the baby is doing well, and that she may safely stay within the mother's body for at least another week without being endangered. Should the baby show signs of distress, it means that the cesarean delivery will take place within a short time, usually within hours. Just in case the cesarean must be accomplished at this time, the mother will be advised to abstain from eating and drinking for 8 hours prior to the test.

If the pattern is good, the mother may go home. She will probably have the test repeated at weekly intervals for as long as is necessary. The objective of giving stress tests to mothers who have special problems is to ensure delivery of the baby at a time that is optimal for *both* the mother and her child. Relaxation breathing exercises will help relieve any nervous tension the mother may have during this test. *The contractions will not cause pain or discomfort.* The sensation is similar to Braxton-Hicks contractions and is felt as a tightening of the uterus.

These tests, singly or in combination with one another, are not totally infallible, but they are better than anything yet devised to make certain that the baby is born healthy and fully matured. In all likelihood, judicious use of these tests during cesarean pregnancies will lead to a reduction in the number of babies born with respiratory distress syndrome and other neonatal problems. Ultrasound, l/s ratio, estriol counts, and nonstress and stress testing are newly developed ways of communicating with the baby before she is born.

CHAPTER 6   SIGNS OF LABOR AND
WHAT TO DO

*H*OW MANY WOMEN are lulled into thinking that because they will deliver by cesarean they are somehow immune to labor? It *can* happen. It may occur weeks before the baby is due, or the night before the scheduled delivery. It does not happen often, but the cesarean mother should be prepared just in case labor does occur spontaneously.

The experience of a woman in the Midwest will illustrate the point. She had seen her doctor in the afternoon. He told her that she was doing "nicely" and that she should check into the hospital the next morning for tests. On the way home from the doctor's office, she began to have what she described as a bad backache. By the time she and her husband arrived home, the ache was localized in her lower abdomen, and felt like menstrual cramps. She curled up on the couch, and put her head on her husband's lap. But she did not call the obstetrician because she didn't want to bother "such a busy man" and because she did not want to call him for something so "trivial" as a few cramps. She thought that if she waited a bit longer, the cramps would go away. When her membranes ruptured and flooded their nice, white contemporary sofa, her husband told her that perhaps she could wait, but he couldn't. He called the doctor. Just over an hour later, she had her baby delivered by cesarean. The doctor later told her that it was a good thing she didn't wait any longer, for her uterine incision from the previous cesarean was "paper thin."

Cesarean parents should know the signs of labor. They are: loss of the mucus plug, bloody show, rupture of the membranes (breaking of the amniotic sac or "bag of waters"), and/or contractions. Panic is not necessary, but the obstetrician should be called immediately, and the expectant mother should abstain from all foods and beverages—including water. If the baby must be delivered within an hour or so, it is safer for her to have an empty stomach.

If you begin having contractions, the way to tell if they are the "real thing" or Braxton-Hicks contractions, the testing contractions which occur during pregnancy, is to stop whatever you are doing and do something else. If you have been lying in bed, get up and walk around. If you have been sitting in a chair, lie down on your left side with your knees slightly bent. Braxton-Hicks contractions are felt in varying intensity and with varying frequency after about the seventh month of pregnancy. If the contractions you are having are of the Braxton-Hicks variety, they will cease or diminish considerably within a few minutes.

THE BENEFITS OF SPONTANEOUS LABOR

What happens if the expectant cesarean mother goes into labor spontaneously days or weeks before the baby is due? Is it dangerous for either her or the baby? Unless labor occurs very prematurely (many weeks or months early), spontaneous labor does not necessarily mean the birth of a premature infant. It is thought that the same hormones which trigger labor may also stimulate the baby's systems and prepare her for life outside the uterus. The usually mild contractions of early labor will probably not be strong enough to rupture the uterus and are not a great threat to either the mother or her baby.

Spontaneous labor is nature's way of telling us that this is the time when the baby should be born. Some doctors (and many parents) do not advocate scheduling elective and repeat cesarean deliveries. They prefer instead to let nature take its course. If labor is truly too early, the mother will go to the hospital where she may be given drugs or alcohol intravenously in sufficient quantities to stop labor. If those measures fail, the baby will be delivered. The premature baby will have the benefits of the skills and technology of the special care nursery where everything possible will be done to help. With modern equipment and techniques, the chances of the premature infant's survival are greatly improved.

If you would like to be permitted to go into labor spontaneously, discuss the possibilities with your obstetrician. Spontaneous labor will save you the long wait in the hospital the night before a scheduled cesarean birth, and will assure you that you have chosen nature's time for the birth. A cesarean birth can take place safely no matter what time of the day or night it is. However, especially in the smaller hospitals, the advantages of scheduling a cesarean delivery are that a full quota of staff will be on duty and ready, and that the cesarean delivery room and all the appropriate equipment and supplies will have been prepared in advance.

IS SUBSEQUENT VAGINAL DELIVERY POSSIBLE?

No discussion of the benefits of spontaneous labor would be complete without exploring the feasibility of a subsequent vaginal delivery. In some instances, it is possible to achieve a successful vaginal delivery after having had one cesarean delivery. The consensus of opinion among American doctors today is that a subsequent vaginal delivery is possible but not probable. The concern is that the strength of labor contractions and the mother's efforts to expel the baby may lead to uterine rupture. If uterine rupture occurs, it means certain death for the unborn baby, and places the mother's life in danger as well. Uterine rupture does not happen frequently. In fact, estimates of the incidence of uterine rupture during delivery is about one percent or less of all births.[1]

Parents who wish to pursue the possibility of a subsequent vaginal delivery (and they are growing in number, as well as in their determination) should of course consult with their obstetricians. Couples who are determined to have at least a trial of labor and attempt a vaginal delivery may have to contact as many as a dozen doctors in their area before finding even one who will consider the proposal. Comparing United States statistics to those in England is revealing. The incidence of cesarean deliveries in England (currently about 5 percent) is far lower than ours, and medical practitioners do not adhere to the American once-a-cesarean-always-a-cesarean rule. In England only 12 percent of all primary cesarean mothers deliver again by repeat cesarean.[2]

Not every woman who wishes to attempt a subsequent vaginal delivery will be able to do so—and not every cesarean mother wishes to try. The cesarean mother who would like to try a vaginal delivery must be carefully screened. Her complete medical history will be taken into account along with the indication for her first delivery by cesarean. What happens very often is that after a trial labor, the woman runs into the same problems she encountered in her first labor. If a woman has had difficulty delivering a seven- or eight-pound baby, it stands to reason that she may have just as much problem delivering a second one of the same size or larger.

Women who are not permitted to attempt a subsequent vaginal delivery, no matter how much they would like to, include: women who have had more than one cesarean; women whose pelvic structure has been proven insufficient; women who have had the classic uterine incision (although this incision is not done very commonly today, there may be a few women whose doctors have had to use the classic up-and-down uterine incision); women with diabetes or other chronic problems; women who show evidence of toxemia;

women whose babies are presenting in a position other than the vertex one (the narrowest part of the head presenting). Some doctors place a further restriction on the potential candidate. For example, some doctors require that at least two years elapse between pregnancies. And all conscientious doctors want their clients to be aware of the risks as well.

Yes, a subsequent vaginal delivery is possible. It is a decision that must be shared by both the parents-to-be and the obstetrician. There is evidence to suggest that the American practice of routinely performing repeat cesarean deliveries may change. A vaginal delivery may have advantages to both the mother and baby. It also carries a certain amount of risk. These must be weighed together before deciding if the potential dangers are worthwhile. Dr. J. Robert McTammany, Chief of Obstetrics at Community General Hospital in Reading, Pennsylvania, voices an opinion shared by other obstetricians, midwives, and maternity personnel, "I have occasionally let previously sectioned mothers deliver vaginally, but it really scares me and I prefer to have them deliver by repeat cesarean. I have very few rigid rules and try always to adapt my technique to the couple and the clinical situation they present."

Two reasons why women may have pursued the possibility of a subsequent vaginal delivery with such vigor are that (1) until very recently, the cesarean procedure was not so much a "birth" as a purely surgical procedure, and (2) until recently, the prevailing attitude seemed to be that something was "wrong" with being unable to deliver vaginally and that the mother who can achieve a vaginal delivery was more like a "real woman." Current attitudes are changing dramatically and rapidly. Emphasis is being placed on a safe, healthy, and emotionally satisfying experience regardless of the method of delivery. If you cannot attempt a vaginal delivery because of medical contraindications or because you cannot find a doctor locally who will go along with the idea, you will probably be temporarily disappointed. You want a healthy baby and a safe delivery for both yourself and your baby—as does the well-intentioned doctor. It is reassuring to know that there is an alternative that can be just as fulfilling, equally exciting and meaningful for you and your husband, and, above all, safe for you and your baby.

CHAPTER 7   HOSPITAL ADMISSION AND
ROUTINES: PREPARING FOR
THE BIRTH

*B*EING ADMITTED to the hospital the afternoon before a scheduled cesarean delivery is not eagerly anticipated by the majority of repeat and elective cesarean mothers. However, a few look forward to this day as a time of rest and relaxation—when dinner is served to them and there are no dishes to do afterwards. For most of us, the time that elapses between 1 or 2 in the afternoon when we are admitted, and 8 or 9 a.m. the next day is a waste of time and money. Cesarean mothers are not sick. They are simply going to have a baby, albeit by appointment. It would be much nicer to be able to spend the afternoon and evening before at home with loved ones, and to sleep in one's own bed. And most of us have no trouble imagining what we could do with the $100 or so that goes for the use of a hospital room which isn't really needed. There is a growing trend in some areas (and it is hoped that it will spread) that allows elective and repeat cesarean mothers to be admitted to the hospital several hours before the delivery, rather than a whole day in advance. This policy makes the occasion seem more like the birth of a baby, and less like a run-of-the-mill, routine surgical procedure. But because that trend is not as yet widespread, this chapter will assume that preadmission the day before is required.

You will be told in advance what time you are expected to check into the hospital. It is usually between noon and 4 p.m. It may be necessary to register at the reception desk, and then wait until you are called into an admitting office to complete paperwork which includes your name, address, social security number, religion, doctor's name, and the person or company responsible for payment of the bill. It will be necessary to sign a release form that states that you understand what type of procedure(s) will be done and that you grant permission for them, as well as for any other previously agreed additional procedures such as tubal ligation or appendectomy. A bracelet will be placed on your wrist, and will remain there until you are discharged. This bracelet is for identification. It contains not only your name, address, and religion, but also your doctor's name, any drug allergies you might have, and a special number that will be the same one that the baby receives on her tags. Then, quite in spite of the fact that you are perfectly all right, it is sometimes required as a matter of preordained hospital policy, that you be taken to your room in a wheelchair.

The purpose of the afternoon admission is for observation and routine preoperative preparations. Vital signs (pulse, blood pressure, and temperature) are taken soon after admission, and every few hours thereafter. Blood samples are drawn so that the lab can do an analysis of your blood type in case transfusion is necessary. Sometimes a test of your respiratory and lung capacity is made. This pulmonary function test requires you to breathe into a tube, similar to a vacuum cleaner hose.

This is also the time when "prepping" of the pubic hair is done. It doesn't hurt, but many women voice the complaint that it is undignified, demeaning, and unnecessary. A total prep is not necessary for cesarean mothers. A partial prep or "poodle cut" is all that is needed—and it is much more comfortable for the woman as the hair grows in. Total preps where every hair from beneath the breasts, between the legs, and up to the tailbone falls victim to the razor are done routinely in some hospitals. Instead of a total prep, a partial prep is much nicer. The partial prep is one in which hair is shaved from the abdomen and pubes—just enough to clear the area where the operation will take place. No hair will be visible when the legs are together. Check in advance to find out what type of prepping is done at your hospital. Your doctor may not know—or even have given the matter much thought. Ask the obstetrician to consider ordering a partial prep. If s/he asks why, you may respond with a question: "How would you like it if it [a full prep] were done to you?"

An anesthesiologist will visit you to inquire about your medical history and your preference for anesthesia. (See the section on anesthesia in this chapter.) Although much of the medical information is on file with your obstetrician, this visit from the anesthesiologist is a good way of double-checking. The medical history will include questions about allergies, physical debilities, weight, and previous surgical experiences. If possible, you may be given a choice of anesthesia (general, spinal, or epidural). Although it is not always possible to have a spinal or epidural (because of your medical history or the doctor's preference) you are free to ask about the various types available to you. If you have any questions, now is the time to ask them. Unless you, too, are an anesthesiologist, you are not expected to know all the hows and whys of anesthesia.

A dietician may come around with a menu for that evening's meal. No matter what your opinion of hospital food (its quality or lack of it), order something and eat it! It's going to be a long time between that meal and your next one. Your body will need to store up vitamins and minerals so that you'll be able to recover more rapidly. If dinner comes and is totally unpalatable, be sure to ask someone to bring something from home or a restaurant. You may feel a little nervous and queasy, too, because of your anticipation of the next day's events. But try to calm yourself and eat something!

Your obstetrician may drop in for a visit during evening

rounds. It is a fact of life that a woman's mind will go blank when the obstetrician walks into the room. All your questions vanish. Just seconds before the doctor came in, you may have been on the verge of tears for some reason or another. "How are you doing?" the doctor asks. Almost automatically, you smile and bravely say, "Just fine, doctor, thank you. Couldn't be better. Thank you for asking. I had some questions but I've forgotten them now." Out goes the doctor, and as soon as s/he has left, you remember what you wanted to say. Always keep a piece of paper and a pen handy while you're in the hospital.

Including dinner, the total amount of time that preoperative routines and visits require can be condensed into about one hour. And it is possible, if you're not prepared, to become bored, restless, or very nervous. Most of the hours that day before are spent in waiting . . . waiting . . . waiting. Chances are that you'll be the only woman on the maternity floor who is still pregnant. All the other mothers are wrapped up in feeding their babies, taking naps, and receiving congratulations from visitors. And there you are, feeling very left out. You may be afraid. It is common to experience anxieties about the health of your baby, the possible danger of anesthesia and surgery, and the responsibilities of caring for a newborn. And if you go for a walk around the floor, you may think your still-pregnant belly stands out like a neon sign. You may even feel a little jealous and depressed. Much of the trepidation you're feeling may be magnified and translated into acute anxiety because, not only are you a little scared, but you may be feeling very trapped. Knowledge of what to expect and how to prepare for this time of waiting, coupled with the support of your mate and the hospital staff, can alleviate these apprehensions.

Prepare in advance for those hours of waiting and wondering. Bring books, write letters, address birth announcements, or finish a project like an embroidered robe for the new baby. Watch television. Make the hospital room more "homey" and personal. Bring pictures of your loved ones, a favorite poster, flowers, or some little treasure from home that makes you feel more secure. Splurge on a long distance phone call to someone you haven't seen in ages. If you keep yourself busy, it will relieve your tensions, and make the time pass more quickly.

Your mate should plan to spend as much of this waiting period with you as possible. Sometimes couples feel inhibited by the hospital atmosphere and the fact that both are tense. Conversation may be stilted—but the important thing is being together. Even if your hospital has 24-hour visiting privileges, your husband will not want to stay all night (unless, of course, there's a bed for him, too—a practice found in a few countries in the world, but not in the United States). Both you and he will need to sleep. He should go home and turn in early. And he should remember to have a "good" breakfast in the morning. Being well hydrated and nourished will make him less apt to become dizzy or faint during the delivery, and will keep him going while waiting for you and the new baby. What he eats isn't important, so long as he has *something* for his stomach juices to nibble on other than each other and the lining of his stomach. He will need this fortification no matter whether he is beside you for the birth, or waiting for you in another part of the hospital.

Speaking of food, you'll be N.P.O. (a Latin abbreviation for nothing by mouth) after midnight. (Women who have never craved a snack in the wee hours of the night may find this is one time in their lives when they become extra thirsty or extra hungry.) If you want to, you may have a light snack around 10 or 11 p.m. Abstinence from food and drink eight hours before delivery is a precautionary measure. Under anesthesia, there is a potential danger of obstructing the breathing passages with vomitus. It is still possible to become nauseated despite the fact that no food has been eaten for many hours prior to the delivery. The potential of this is reduced by abstaining from all foods and beverages at least eight hours before the birth takes place.

Sometime that evening, the nurse may offer you a sleeping pill. Although most medications of this type are prohibited during pregnancy, this is one time when a sleeping tablet may be welcomed. The hospital is strange and noisy. You are probably at least a little tense. You'll need a good night's rest. If you think that the sleeping pill will help, then by all means take it. It will not hurt the baby, since it will have been assimilated and metabolized by your body hours before the baby is born.

Some mothers refuse the sleeping pill—and it is their right to do so if they wish. Sometimes the pills don't work right away, sometimes they don't work at all, and sometimes in spite of the pill, the mother may awaken during the night and need someone to talk with. The floor nurses should be willing to spend some time with the mother, if doing nothing more than listening to her. In fact, if the maternity floor is fairly quiet and unbusy that night, the nurses may enjoy a conversation. Having someone to share even a few minutes with, if you need it, will reduce your anxieties.

The standard of requiring all elective cesarean mothers to be admitted to the hospital the afternoon before delivery has its basis in medical tradition, and, in special cases, good medical practice. It is not always necessary, and sometimes disadvantageous (particularly for the mother who is already anxious about leaving older children at home when she has never been separated from them before). In the meantime, educating cesarean parents in all phases of pregnancy and birth, and giving them prior knowledge of and suggestions for dealing with the "night-before-blues" will make the experience better and less anxiety producing.

ANESTHESIA

An *anesthesiologist* is a doctor who has had special training in the field of anesthesia. S/he decides the type and amount of anesthesia to be given and is able to administer it independently. An *anesthetist* is a highly trained nurse who continues to monitor the patient *after* an anesthesiologist has administered the anesthetic. Anesthetists are not permitted to decide which type is to be used nor administer it without the supervision of an anesthesiologist. These two terms are often confusing to the lay person.

Three types of anesthesia are used for cesarean childbirth: spinal, epidural, and general. With spinals and epidurals, mothers are awake and aware for their babies' births. Pain is totally eliminated although some minor sensation may be experienced. With general anesthesia, the mother is "put to sleep" and is unaware of what is happening until an hour or more after delivery. The type of anesthesia used will depend on several factors:

1. The mother's medical history.
2. The preferences of her doctor and/or the anesthesia department. Trends in obstetric anesthesia are subject to changes in medical "fashion." It is possible to have had general anesthesia with a previous delivery, and then be given a spinal for a subsequent birth. There is a current debate among medical professionals over the renewed interest in general anesthesia for cesarean deliveries. Some health care professionals who favor general anesthesia cite the fact that it *may* reduce the possibility of *hypotension* and thus be better for the mother. *Hypotension* is the condition that may develop as the result of a reduction in the patient's blood pressure that occurs (if it's going to) shortly after anesthesia has been administered. The mother, especially if she is tense or fearful, may become dizzy or nauseated. Additional oxygen or medication can relieve temporary feelings of dizziness or nausea and are a small price to pay for being able to see, hear, and touch one's baby within seconds of birth. If there is a real danger associated with spinal or epidural anesthetic (because of medical contraindications), it should be discussed openly and honestly with the prospective mother before she makes her decision. No mother wants to jeopardize her life or her baby's.

Sometimes the type of anesthesia depends on who is available in the anesthesia department when the cesarean takes place. Smaller community hospitals, unlike major medical facilities, do not always keep round-the-clock teams of anesthesiologists on duty. Therefore the person called in for a cesarean may greatly influence what type is given.

I feel (and other parents and health care professionals join me in this view) that parents should be allowed a choice of anesthesia whenever possible. When there is a choice, parents should be permitted a voice in the decision.

3. Regional bias. The type of anesthesia used for cesarean deliveries (and other operations) sometimes depends on the geographic location of the hospital. An example of "regional bias" is a northern New England hospital that uses general anesthesia routinely. In Boston, one hospital does at least 50 percent of all cesarean deliveries with spinal anesthesia and the remainder with general anesthesia. Another maternity center uses spinal anesthesia for at least 90 percent of the cesarean deliveries that take place there. General anesthesia is used only if there is a medical contraindication, or if the mother insists on it.

4. Time element. Some emergency cesareans really are "emergency emergencies." In such cases, there may be no choice as to which type of anesthesia is used because of the dire necessity of "getting the baby out" as quickly as possible. This situation is beyond the mother's control. The prime consideration is delivering the baby as quickly and as safely as possible, and, if the quickest, safest way is with general anesthesia, it will have to be used. The baby's life is at stake.

5. The final and most important consideration is the mother herself. For a primary (first-time) emergency cesarean delivery, the mother may be exhausted after a trying labor and ask to be given general anesthesia. She may be afraid that there will be additional stress or pain with a spinal or epidural. Because mothers-to-be are not always well-versed with how a cesarean

takes place, they may think that they will hear, see, or feel something "awful." There are also a few women who are told, or suspect, that their babies' lives are endangered, or who dread the thought of seeing a baby born who is deformed. They may use general anesthesia as a sort of self-protection to avoid knowing what happens to them and their babies until they are better able to cope.

By and large, most mothers want to see their babies at birth. Any initial misgivings or fears can be overcome with support and information from the mother's obstetrician, her anesthesiologist, her nurses, and her husband. With education and empathy come confidence: the cesarean mother will know what to expect and how to cope effectively without panic. Being awake for the baby's birth enables the mother to initiate the maternal-infant bonding processes and to rejoice in the baby's arrival.

General Anesthesia. General anesthesia can be given either by placing a mask over the mother's nose and mouth or inserting a needle into her arm. With either method, the mother-to-be becomes unconscious within a few seconds. She will remember nothing until an hour or more after delivery when she groggily awakens. In emergency cesarean deliveries which take place after a trying labor and/or the use of scopolamine (an amnesia-producing drug), women sometimes report that they awoke thinking they were still in labor. Some of these mothers found it hard to believe that their babies had been born, especially if they had also been separated from them for many hours.

The myth that all cesareans must be performed with general anesthesia is persistent and perpetuated partially by contemporary old wives' tales and partially by the lack of information with which cesarean parents have had to contend. It is difficult to make an intelligent decision based on myth and misinformation. When a mother chooses to have general anesthesia, one of her reasons (in fact, the primary one) may be fear: fear of the unknown, fear of possible pain, or the trauma of a previous cesarean birth which makes the thought of being awake anathema to her.

Another reason why some women have general anesthesia is that they are unaware of the alternatives. If the mother has had an opportunity to discuss her anxieties with someone who is able to relate to her experiences, it is not surprising to have her change her mind and ask for a spinal or epidural, rather than general anesthesia. The anesthesiologist is of course a prime source of information and support, but unfortunately, most expectant mothers do not meet with an anesthesiologist until the night before they are to deliver. Therefore, the responsibility of informing parents of the options lies with the obstetrician who sees the mother throughout pregnancy. The mother should feel free to ask questions of her doctor as they come up, and, it is hoped, have her fears set to rest. Also, the support and empathy that another woman or another cesarean mother is able to give are often an added bonus.

Spinals and Epidurals. Spinals and epidurals share the benefit of allowing mothers to be awake, aware, and comfortable for the birth. They reduce the potential negative effects of general anesthesia, which may sometimes cross the placenta and depress the baby's systems. Although spinals are more commonly used than epidurals, the type given depends on many things including your doctor's preference, the hospital's location, and preexisting medical conditions such as blood pressure or severe back problems that would make it difficult, if not impossible, to successfully administer these anesthetics.

Both spinals and epidurals are administered to the patient's back. The epidural takes effect more slowly than the spinal, and additional medication is given during the delivery as necessary to keep the mother comfortable by means of a catheter (a thin tube) which is kept in place during the delivery. The spinal is given by means of injecting a small quantity of medication in the back just once. It is done just a few minutes before the obstetrician is ready to deliver the baby. Both create a temporary paralysis (numbing) from the chest to the tips of the toes. There is usually no sensation whatsoever, but the mother may feel pressure as the baby is actually being delivered. Pressure, pulling, or tugging sensations, which herald the baby's imminent arrival, are discussed in more detail in Chapter 8, Birthday!

Other Forms of Anesthesia. Although there are other forms of anesthesia, they are not widely accepted or used in the United States. Acupuncture is frequently used in China; Shirley MacLaine's film *China: The Other Half of the Sky* shows a cesarean birth taking place with acupuncture as the sole means of anesthesia. The mother is smiling, eating bits of fruit fed to her by a nurse, and waves at the camera. Acupuncture has been used for at least one cesarean birth in the United States.

Some experimentation with hypnosis has been done in this country. A film produced primarily for physicians shows a Midwestern obstetrician and a cesarean mother who is having her third cesarean delivery under hypnosis. It is obvious that the woman and her doctor have worked closely in preparation for the delivery. During the delivery, the mother sings as a means of taking her mind away from what is happening. The doctor suggests that the room is very warm—despite the fact that is is quite cool. The woman is told to open her eyes and look at her baby before she is again placed in a "trance" so that suturing can be done. In an interview soon after the delivery, she remembers no pain, but she does recall that the delivery room was very warm and that she wanted a cool drink to make herself more comfortable.

As anesthetic alternatives, acupuncture and hypnosis are interesting to note, and do emphasize the fact that mind over matter often is an essential key to the reduction of discomfort.

Making the Choice. My intention is not to persuade women to have anesthesia that will permit them to be awake for the birth of their babies if they are truly unwilling. Before making the decision (when there *is* a choice) it is advisable to weigh the pros and cons and to consider the possible benefits and risks

of each type of anesthesia. A woman who is deeply fearful
will probably be better off having general anesthesia. She may
be afraid of hearing or seeing unpleasant things. General anesthesia *may* (but not necessarily) cross the placenta faster than
other types, and thus depress the baby's systems. The real
benefits of regional anesthetics are often enumerated in human,
rather than medical, terms. The cesarean delivery *is* the birth
of a baby. Many women wish to participate in the birth, to
feel a part of the goings on. This can be done with spinal or
epidural anesthesia. The cesarean mother will be unable to
control the situation and expel the baby by her own efforts,
but she *will* be able to hear her baby's first cries, and will
see her infant within seconds or minutes of birth. She is often
able to establish eye contact with her infant within a short
time after birth, and may also be able to touch the baby with
her face, kiss the infant, and reassure herself that the infant
is well. This promotes the mother-infant bonding and attachment processes, and may help the mother feel more like a
"real" mother sooner. This does not mean that women who
have general anesthesia are "bad" mothers, or that they may
turn out to be less "motherly." What it does mean is simple:
seeing a newborn within seconds and being both comfortable
and awake for the birth *may* make it easier for the mother to
finalize her pregnancy and initiate her role of parent. If you
have general anesthesia because of medical conditions (such as
previous back injury or blood pressure problems), or because
it is the only type of anesthesia available where you deliver,
or because you choose to, then be assured that the doctor will
work as quickly as possible to deliver the baby before the
anesthesia crosses the placenta. If you are highly motivated
(which you probably are), you will relate well to your baby no
matter what type of anesthesia is given.

The important thing is for you to feel comfortable—both
physically and mentally—with whatever type of anesthesia you
have. If you have been too apprehensive to ask for a spinal or

epidural, perhaps you would like to reconsider. A discussion with your obstetrician will give you an accurate picture of what your particular situation is. Each woman, each pregnancy, each baby, each doctor, and each hospital are different. The type of anesthesia used for a prior delivery or how your friends had babies is not as important as knowing that the decision is one you and your doctor have made after careful consideration. You should feel confident and relaxed about the type of anesthesia to be used. Your physical comfort, your baby's well-being, and your emotional satisfaction are the primary concerns.

HOW TO MAKE THE ADMINISTRATION OF ANESTHESIA EASIER

With an emergency cesarean, there is not usually enough time to worry about the type of anesthesia used. During subsequent pregnancies, however, cesarean mothers may be very apprehensive about anesthesia. One of their anxieties is the actual administration of the anesthetic. To make the administration of a spinal or epidural easier, for both you and the anesthesiologist, here are some suggestions on how to cope effectively.

Administration of anesthesia requires just a few minutes. During this period you will want to be as relaxed, comfortable, and confident as possible.

If the baby's father is to be present for the birth, he may be asked to wait outside the delivery room until after you have been given the anesthesia. If he is in the room, he may have to sit off to the side for this procedure. While preparations are being made, a way to break tension is to converse with the anesthesiologist, your obstetrician, the delivery room nurses, or your husband. You may be jokingly asked what color anesthesia you want: blue for a boy, or pink for a girl. The obstetrician will be in the room by this time, because s/he will want to begin the delivery very soon after the anesthesia has taken effect. It is helpful to establish eye contact with someone in the room. You're going to have a baby, and seeing someone's face is much more reassuring than staring at the ceiling tiles or the drape in front of you.

You will be told to turn on your side, and bring your knees up to your chin. This is certainly not a difficult request under most circumstances, but there you are with a big "lump" of a tummy in the way. Most pregnant women haven't even been able to see their toes in the last month or two, so having to pull your knees all the way up to your chin will require a bit of effort. What the anesthesiologist is really asking you to do is to flex (bend) as much as possible. Operating tables are notoriously narrow (so that the obstetrician and the assisting physician are able to stand as close as possible to the area of the incision). Don't be afraid. Those tables are wide enough to accommodate even a 300-pound patient. You will be assisted by the nurse and anesthesiologist. One of the nurses will help you turn, and will probably aid you by lifting your knees and supporting your body.

After your knees are flexed, you will be asked to arch your back toward the anesthesiologist. As long as you are aware of what is happening and why, this part should not be difficult. Discipline and relaxation breathing techniques will help. Think of your body as a *rainbow* and arch *toward* the anesthesiologist. Your initial reaction may be to pull away from the doctor, who will by now be "painting" your back with a cool antiseptic solution. (For some reason, it often seems as though everything in a hospital is cool.) Arching serves to separate and make more visible the bones of the spine, and thus makes it easier for the doctor to administer the anesthesia. After the antiseptic solution goes on, you may feel a stinging sensation as a novocaine-like drug is injected. The important thing to remember is that this part takes just a few minutes. Being aware of what is happening and knowing that it will be over soon will help you to cope effectively and comfortably.

Some anesthesiologists encourage mothers to "arch your

back like a mad cat." A mad cat is a tense cat, and because relaxation is important for this step, the image of a rainbow is really preferable because it is more soothing.

(There are many reasons why pregnant women are advised to keep their weight within reasonable limits. One of them is that the anesthesiologist may have a harder time finding the "landmarks" of the spine and the introduction of anesthesia may take longer than is necessary. Also, if there is a thick layer of fat between the abdomen and the uterus, it will take longer for the obstetrician to reach the uterus and then to suture all those extra layers.)

Although you may have had to wait for the delivery room to be free, the doctors to arrive, and the room to be set up, once the anesthesia has been given, it will be just 5 or 10 minutes until your baby is born. From here on in, the team-work and precision of the staff, and the eagerness of seeing, hearing, and touching your baby should be comforting—and, it is hoped, a fulfilling, enjoyable occasion.

TYPES OF SKIN INCISIONS

Generally when parents talk about incisions, they are referring to the skin incision only. Actually the obstetrician needs to make a series of incisions, not just one, to reach the uterus. The skin incision is the only visible one, and is often referred to by cesarean mothers as "the scar." There are two types of skin incisions. The *classic incision* is a midline abdominal incision that extends from just below the navel to the top of the pubic bone. The *transverse* or *lower segment incision,* often referred to as a "bikini cut," goes from side to side just above the pubic bone. Its cosmetic advantage is that once the pubic hair regrows, it is barely visible.

Which type of skin incision you have will depend on:

1. The time element involved. Sometimes doctors use a classic incision for an emergency cesarean because it may save time.

2. Your doctor's preference. Some doctors feel more comfortable using one type of incision rather than the other.

3. Sometimes the mother's preference. This is not always possible, especially if time is of the essence.

In recent years, the lower segment incision has gained popularity among medical professionals and mothers. If yours is a repeat cesarean, the new incision will be made at the same location as the old one. If your scar is thick, the doctor will remove it. In other words, contrary to contemporary myth, the repeat cesarean mother will not have plus signs, anchors, or crosses emblazoned upon her abdomen no matter how many cesarean deliveries she has. This misconception is very widespread, especially among mothers who have not had babies in several years. They erroneously assume that because the transverse "bikini cut" is now so popular, that they will have to have two incisions instead of one. Using the same location for subsequent incisions reduces the possibility of their weakening and perhaps rupturing.

It is also important to note that no matter which type of skin incision one has, the uterine incision is almost always transverse (horizontal, from side to side). Today, it is known that the classic uterine incision (vertical, up and down) may weaken the uterus. So, as a general rule, almost all of today's cesarean deliveries take place with a lower segment uterine incision.

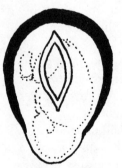

**Classic Uterine
Incision**

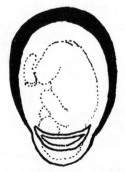

**Lower Segment or Transverse
Uterine Incision**

CHAPTER 8 BIRTHDAY!

*A*T LAST! This is the day!
All the waiting, wondering, and worrying will soon be past.
Finally the baby you have been carrying for nine months will
be revealed. You will be able to see, hold, love, cuddle, and
kiss your baby. You will soon know if it is a boy or a girl. You
will be able to see if the baby has inherited your hair, your
husband's eyes, or grandma's nose. But before all these things
can happen, you and your baby will undergo a series of complex steps. The quality of the birth experience, the way you,
the parents, will relate to the baby, and how soon you recover
will depend on what happens during the baby's birth. If you
feel relaxed, confident, and informed, this will be a beautiful
day for you, and a time in which the roots of love are planted.

There should be time for you to take a shower before
donning a hospital gown called a "johnny." This is one of
those garments that is always too big, ties in the back, and is
anything but fashionable—but it is efficient. Your husband
should be allowed to come to the hospital several hours or so
before the scheduled delivery. He may walk into your room
carrying the morning paper, and hiding behind a self-conscious
smile which betrays his air of assurance. He, too, is feeling a
little nervous and eager. This morning is, for both of you,
a little like a surprise party that you found out about in
advance. You won't be surprised by the party, but you will be
delighted with the present.

Although each person's experience is unique, the following is a general outline of what you can expect:

Usually, the mother-to-be is given an enema the morning of the delivery. Although no one has ever been recorded as being excited and happy with this prospect, it is nothing to get upset about. Think of it in terms of the future: emptying the bowels this morning will mean that the new mother won't have to do so shortly after the birth, when she feels uncomfortable enough with the stitches and other postoperative discomforts. Sitting on a bedpan within a few hours after delivery is anything but pleasant.

A Foley catheter (thin tube) will be inserted into the urethra (the duct by which urine is discharged from the bladder). Catheterization can take place in the mother's room, or shortly after she has been taken to the delivery room. Insertion is not painful, but some women report that it can be a little uncomfortable. If you find yourself tense or if the insertion is uncomfortable, relaxation breathing should help. Usually it takes just a few seconds. Once the catheter is properly in place, you probably won't feel it at all and will forget that it's there. How long the catheter remains in place depends on the doctor's orders and the mother's condition. About 24 hours is typical, although it may remain in place for several days. The Foley catheter has two purposes. The immediate one is that it drains the bladder and keeps it compressed and out of the doctor's way as the baby is delivered. The other is that it eliminates the mother's need to urinate into a bedpan or get out of bed to go to the bathroom. Occasionally an infection will develop, but infection is not common, and usually occurs only if the catheter has been in place for many days.

Some doctors order a tranquilizer to be injected shortly before the mother is taken from her room to the delivery room. This is one occasion when it may be advisable *not* to accept this medication. (Your body will tell you if you should take or refuse it.) If the mother-to-be is especially tense, then she may prefer it. If she has composed herself, it is not necessary, and may in fact, have a deleterious effect on the baby. Drugs such as Nembutal and Valium are seldom if ever given to a laboring woman an hour or so before delivery since drugs pass quickly through the placenta and into the baby. Cesarean babies who have not had the beneficial stimulation of labor may be unnecessarily "zapped" and "slowed down" if tranquilizers are used shortly before birth. Neither the mother's body nor the baby's will have time to metabolize and assimilate this medication. Cesarean babies do not need this extra burden. Rather than take a chance of depressing the baby's system, cesarean mothers may wish to refuse this medication. If you decide that you really need it, however, you should not feel guilty about accepting it.

The best preoperative "tranquilizer" for a cesarean mother is the presence of the baby's father to support and reassure her and the confidence that comes from knowing what to expect and how to cope calmly and effectively.

In a few hospitals, the cesarean mother-to-be is allowed to walk from her room to a labor room or directly into the delivery room holding hands with the baby's father if she likes. Both a nurse and the baby's father accompany her. She is not "ill" in the conventional sense, and if she has not been dosed with a tranquilizer, it helps to make the experience seem more like a "birth" and less like a "standard surgical procedure." If walking is not permitted, a wheelchair rather than a stretcher may be used.

Whether she is taken to the cesarean delivery room (or, in some hospitals, the regular operating suite) on a stretcher, in a wheelchair, or allowed to walk there, there will be sufficient time for the mother and father to share a few moments together, encouraging each other, hugging and kissing—or crying. The tears that come just before delivery are often a combination of happiness and nervous release. If the father is not permitted to be present for the birth, this is when the couple will have to part. He will be asked to wait in the fathers' waiting room, the lobby, or he may sit in an empty labor room or in the hallway just outside the delivery suite. Hospital policy will determine where he waits. It is hoped that the father will be able to rejoice in the birth, to be with the mother, either sitting or standing beside her. Even if he is allowed to share in the birth, many hospitals will ask him to wait outside for a few minutes while preoperative preparations are made, and anesthesia given. Sometimes this waiting period is lengthy. Each doctor, each nurse, and every piece of equipment must be in place before the delivery can begin. Sometimes obstetricians are late. Sometimes the cesarean delivery room is not free when the birth is scheduled. (If the father is asked to wait while the preparations are being made, it's a good idea to ask approximately how long the wait will be. Don't panic and think that they have started without you, or forgotten to call you in. It may take as long as 30 minutes to "set up.")

In the delivery room, the mother will be the center of a flurry of activity. Once on the operating table, there is much to be done. Although the order of events may vary, these are some of things that will happen:

One arm will have a blood pressure cuff wrapped around it, so that your blood pressure can be monitored as often as needed. In the other arm, the anesthesiologist will start an i.v. (intravenous). The intravenous will keep the mother hydrated and nourished during the procedure, and perhaps for hours or days thereafter. The i.v. is also an important emergency route should additional drugs or blood transfusion be necessary. The amount of blood loss during a cesarean is usually only about a pint. If there is greater bleeding, blood will be administered through this i.v. Starting the i.v. before the delivery begins will make the mother less apt to become hypotensive. Her blood pressure will remain more stable if she has the benefits of extra liquids in advance of delivery, and she will probably not experience some of the side effects associated with anesthesia.

The arm with the blood pressure cuff will be placed at your side. Sometimes it remains free; at other hospitals, it may be tucked in. Many women envision their arms as being strapped and practically chained to the table. This is not true. Often the restraint consists of a sheet placed under her back, and brought up around her arm, to be tucked in again at her side. When both arms are secured, it lessens the danger of contaminating the sterile field (the body area to be operated on, that is, your abdomen).

As soon as the anesthesia has been given, and we will assume in this instance it is a spinal, the mother will be quickly turned on her back. [For types of anesthesia and how to make the administration easier, see page 82.] Turning her quickly will serve to spread the anesthesia equally. Although she may be unaware of it, the operating table will be tilted slightly to the side, usually the left, to enable the doctor to be closer to the site of the incisions, and to take the pressure of the relaxed uterus off the vena cava (the major vein which runs from the lower extremities). If cesarean mothers could see what happens in a few minutes after the anesthesia has been given, they would see that the abdomen relaxes and spreads out slightly. (It is similar to what happens when a bowl of gelatin is unmolded properly.) If the full weight of the uterus and fetus are not taken off the vena cava, it will interfere with the mother's circulation, and may produce minor difficulties in breathing, shortness of breath, and/or a lowering of the blood pressure, which may cause nausea or dizziness.

After the anesthesia has been administered, a number of things are done and done so quickly that the mother may be unaware of them. Little disks will be placed on her chest, with wires running to an electrocardiograph (e.k.g.). We have all seen medical shows which give this machine a great deal of attention. A little line goes up and down, with more or less rhythmic bleeps emitted. Quite frequently in "real life," the "stickers" (the little sensory disks which are placed on the mother's chest) become unstuck. And, e.k.g.'s have been known to malfunction. When this happens, you (if you are at all aware of the "bleeps") may wonder what has happened. You've seen enough television shows to know that when the bleep becomes constant, or when the line goes flat (instead of showing a series of peaks and valleys), the person is dead.

While having a cesarean, more than one woman has been known to think she has died when the e.k.g. machine has malfunctioned. There she is thinking, "Oh, my God. This is awful. Here I am dead and I can still hear and see." If you can hear it, if you can see what is going on, if you *think* you've died, you haven't. It just means that the machine went on the fritz.

An anesthesia screen is also put into place just below the mother's neck. Her gown is draped over it, and is covered by another sterile sheet. Its major purpose is to keep the mother from breathing on and thus contaminating the sterile field, but it blocks her view so that all she will be able to see are the areas on her side, the drape in front of her, and the ceiling above. It is a very limited view. If you want to see what is happening below the drapes, it is sometimes possible to look into the overhead light. Someday, perhaps, women who wish to watch their babies born by cesarean will be able to do so in mirrors such as the ones used for vaginal deliveries. Ten or fifteen years ago, using a mirror for vaginal deliveries seemed as "outrageous" and "farfetched" an idea as contemporary cesarean mothers asking for one. The refusal of a mirror is often well-intentioned, but it is an option to which cesarean mothers are entitled. Women who don't want to see what is happening won't ask for a mirror, and a woman who has requested a mirror and becomes uneasy with what she sees can avert her eyes. If a cesarean mother has prior knowledge of what to expect and the desire to watch her baby born, there is no reason to deny her a mirror.

Also as part of the preparations made for the delivery, a nurse or the obstetrician will apply an antiseptic solution to the mother's abdomen and partway down her legs. It has a rusty, iodine color, and to the uninitiated it may look as though the abdomen has been painted with blood. Sterile drapes, often made of paper, are then placed over the entire lower portion of the mother's body, leaving only the area immediately surrounding the incision site visible.

If nausea, dizziness, or vomiting are to occur, they will

probably happen within a few minutes after the anesthesia has been given. Nausea, dizziness, or vomiting *may* happen no matter how long it has been since you last ate, no matter how quickly you are turned, no matter how much the table is tilted, and no matter how calm, cool and collected you are! It is something that happens *sometimes*. It does not happen to everyone. Panic is the worst reaction to have. If it happens to you, the *first* thing to do is to tell the anesthesiologist, who will give you a little tray to throw up in, and/or may give you additional intravenous medication if necessary.

Oxygen is an excellent way to combat these feelings of nausea or dizziness. The oxygen mask may be made of clear plastic material, or of black, "funny-smelling" rubber. The "funny" smell may come from the rubber itself, or from traces of the odor of other gases for which it has been used. The mask is sterilized before each use, but the odd smell may linger. Don't panic and think that the anesthesiologist is trying to pull a fast switch and knock you out. When the mask is in place, take big, deep breaths of oxygen for as long as you need it. Lots of extra oxygen will bring almost immediate relief.

When all these preparations have been completed, it is time for the birth of your baby. First-time, emergency cesarean mothers who have been in labor for many hours may have little recollection of just how long the actual delivery took. Repeat cesarean mothers may be acutely aware of each second that passes. It is comforting and useful to know that the amount of time between the introduction of anesthesia and the delivery of the new baby is usually just 5 to 10 minutes. How long it takes is a matter of the doctor's speed (some doctors are real "roadrunners" and take just a few minutes to reach the baby; others, no less skillful, may take a little longer); how heavy the mother is (it takes extra time to cut through layer after layer of fat); what position the baby is in; what type of anesthesia is used and what the indication is for the delivery ("emergency" emergencies such as abruptio placenta necessitate the greatest speed while other indications

may permit the doctor to work somewhat more slowly).
Generally, though, it takes 5 to 10 minutes. The doctor will
work as quickly as possible no matter what the circumstances.
It is necessary to deliver the baby rapidly to reduce the potentially dangerous effects of anesthesia to the fetus. After the
baby has been delivered, the pace can be more leisurely, less
pressured.

If this is a repeat cesarean, the new incision will be made
at the site of the old one. The incision is then retracted (pulled
back) to reveal the layers beneath the skin. There are layers of
subcutaneous fat, the fascia (a tough membrane), abdominal
muscles, and the peritoneum (a thin membrane protecting the
abdominal cavity and the organs therein). Once these layers
have been incised, the doctor can see the uterus, which is a
royal purple color. An incision is then made in the wall of the
uterus. The transverse (from side to side) incision, which is
made in the lower part of the uterus, is surprisingly short.
Three or four inches across is about average. As the uterus
is opened, the amniotic fluid may gush out, showering the
doctors. If the amniotic sac is intact, the doctor will pierce
it, and suction the fluid out. At this time there may be a
whooshing noise which sounds almost like the little tube the
dentist places in your mouth to extract fluids. When you hear
this noise, it means that it's almost time for the baby to be
born.

When retracted, the 3- or 4-inch opening in the uterus is
about the same size as a fully dilated cervix (10 centimeters).
To remove the baby through this relatively small opening, it is
sometimes necessary for the obstetrician or the assisting physician to exert pressure on the top of the uterus. Some women
report that they can feel this pressure or pulling. It is not painful, but the surprise element of it may cause a woman to
panic, to think that the anesthesia has not taken effect
properly. If it happens to you, don't panic. First tell the
doctor that you are having this sensation. Second, relaxation
and/or dissociative breathing may help. Third, and *most*

important, remember that if you do feel this pressure, it is a *good* sign. It means that your baby will be born within a few seconds or minutes at most. This sensation heralds your baby's birth.

How can you tell if it's going to happen to you? You can't. Primary, emergency cesarean mothers, especially those who deliver by cesarean after labor has begun, may be exhausted. "I was so tired out the first time, they could have run over me with a Mack truck and I wouldn't have known the difference" is a typical reaction. The second time around, the cesarean mother has probably been scheduled for delivery. She is not fatigued as a result of labor, and her senses may be especially keen.

Before, during, and after the birth, it is vitally necessary, comforting, and helpful for the doctors and nurses to talk *with* the mother—especially if the father is not beside her. The mother should be asked what *she* wants to talk about. Some mothers prefer a running commentary given by the obstetrician, "I've made the skin incision. . . . Now I've reached the peritoneum. . . . I can see the uterus now. . . . Here comes the baby's head, now the shoulders. . . . Just a few more seconds and we'll see if this little one is a boy or a girl. . . ."

It would be nice to be able to say that the days of doctors and nurses talking about the mother, rather than with and to her, are gone. It would be even nicer to be able to say that doctors are no longer indulging in conversations with each other about fishing trips, French restaurants, or Colonial architecture. Unfortunately, such a statement would be fallacious.

The mother should be made to feel as though she is a woman giving birth, rather than a hunk of flesh being operated on. This is the birth of a baby, not a rap session at a country club sauna. The mother and her baby should be the only topics of discussion, unless the mother herself wants to talk about other things. Talking between doctors during surgery is often a way for them to relieve tension. If the mother has had general anesthesia, it really doesn't matter what they say to each other, but when general anesthesia is used, a nurse or the baby's father should hold the mother's hand and reassure her until she is asleep. The mother who is awake for the birth of her baby should not be degraded and demoralized. (One mother said, "For all the attention they paid to me, they could just as well have unscrewed my head from my torso, and taken only my trunk into the delivery room." Another woman commented, "I felt just like the woman in a magic show. My head was at one end of a box, and my feet were sticking out the other end. It seemed as though there were miles in between my head and my body.")

Conversing with the mother will relieve the doctors' and her tension, and will make her feel like a woman giving birth, rather than an incidental object in the room. If the father is present for the birth, he can comfort the mother, describe to her what is happening, and reassure her that all is well.

The size of the delivery room is sometimes a surprise to parents, who are familiar only with the huge amphitheaters pictured on television. Large teaching hospitals do have huge delivery rooms, with balconies for observation, but most community hospital delivery rooms (whether they are regular operating rooms or a special cesarean room within the delivery suite) are far smaller. The small size of the cesarean delivery room is one factor taken into consideration by some hospitals when considering the possibility of allowing fathers in for the birth. Almost without exception, there will always be room for one more, very important person: the father.

The father is required to wear a scrub suit, mask, and cap and will be asked to either sit or stand beside the mother's head. If he is seated, his view will be almost as limited as the mother's, and it will be the doctor who announces the arrival and sex of the baby. Fathers who are allowed to stand can see and will want to make this announcement.

If the baby is lying in the normal position (head down), the top of the baby's head will be the first thing the doctor sees, once the uterus has been opened. If the baby is in the breech position, the buttocks are the first visible body part. When the uterus is open, the doctor will reach inside with her/his hands and pull the baby out. Forceps are occasionally used, but these are employed less often nowadays. As soon as the baby's head is out, the doctor or assistant will suction the mucus from the baby's nose and mouth. At this point, the parents may hear the baby's first cries. And what a beautiful sound! If the baby has a large quantity of mucus, the first cry may sound more like a gurgle. Hearing that cry, the first question any parent will ask is, "What is it? Is it a boy or a girl?" If the doctor's reply is, "I don't know yet," the parents may think that the baby is a hermaphrodite—unless they know there is a short period between delivery of the baby's head and its body. When the umbilical cord is long enough, the doctor may hold the baby up for the mother to see, while the cord is still attached and the baby is all wet and covered with vernix (a creamy, protective substance). This sight will be just as every parent pictures it. It will look just like the films and photos of babies who are delivered vaginally, and who are shown to the mother a split second after it has emerged. Brand new babies are bluish in color. As the oxygen reaches the body, the baby will gradually "pink up." Because of their distance from the heart, the last part of the baby's body to turn pink will be her hands and feet. The newborn may react to the birth in a manner similar to a shadow-boxer, as she uncurls from the fetal position. This is both good and healthy. After nine months in the mother's warm, dark, watery world, the bright lights of the delivery room, the relative coolness of its temperature, and the initial "shock" of suddenly having to function and breathe on her own stimulate her body. As soon as the baby has been delivered, the umbilical cord will be clamped and cut.

After holding the baby up for the mother to see, (and the father, too, if he is there) the baby will be placed in the arms of a nurse or pediatrician. Some nurses bring the naked baby immediately over to the mother to see. Then the baby is quickly placed in a specially equipped basinette. There she will be placed under warming lights (similar to the type which keep food hot in restaurants); additional oxygen will be given to her and mucus suctioned from her nose and mouth. (Cesarean babies, because they have not been squeezed through the birth canal, often have more mucus than babies delivered vaginally.) The additional oxygen given through a tiny mask will ensure an adequate supply of this vitally important substance. Her Apgar score, a quick, simple rating of the baby's reflexes (see chart below) will be taken. Apgar scores are taken at one and five minutes after birth. The rating system was developed by Dr. Virginia Apgar as a standardized way to record the infants' reflexes. A score of 8 or higher indicates a healthy baby. Mild problems may be present in babies with an Apgar of between 5 and 7. Below 5 means that the baby will need immediate, intensive care.

APGAR RATING SYSTEM

Sign: Score:	0	1	2
Color	blue, pale	body pink, limbs blue	completely pink
Respiratory effort	absent	slow, irregular, weak cry	strong cry
Heart rate	absent	slow, less than 100	over 100
Muscle tone	limp	some flexation of limbs	active movement
Reflex response to flicking foot	absent	facial grimace	cry

The mother and father have waited a long time for the baby to be born. This is the moment they have anticipated eagerly and occasionally agonized over. Seeing a new baby is an extraordinarily beautiful, awe-inspiring, spiritual sight. This is why it is important for the doctor or nurse to hold the baby for viewing by the mother within seconds of delivery, and why it is infinitely preferable for the baby care unit to be placed within the mother's sight.

To understand just how important this is, doctors and nurses should picture themselves in the mother's place. Some hospitals are now holding informal consciousness-raising sessions where one of the staff members actually lies on the delivery table, with an anesthesia screen in place. For dramatic effect, two other people, playing the role of the obstetrician and the assistant physician, carry on a conversation which might go something like this:

First Person: Say, Joe, I wanted to tell you about a nice little French restaurant Marilyn and I went to last night. The food was just great.

Second Person: Oh, yeah? What did you have? I'll hold that retractor.

First Person: Knife. . . . Give me the knife. Frogs' legs. Marilyn had snails.

Second Person: Hmmm. That's nice. I haven't had frogs' legs in a long time. How were they?

First Person: Whoooops! Let's get that bleeder. . . . Not enough garlic for my taste. I'm having a little trouble here. Pressure, give me fundal pressure.

Second Person: I've got the bulb. Here. Clamp the cord.

First Person: Hey, nurse, take the kid. Joe, get that cord blood.

Is that any way to handle the most significant event in a woman's life? Doctors and nurses might also "Try sometime putting your head close to a woman having a cesarean birth. See how restricted her visual field is and listen to the noises: the rustle of paper drapes, the snip of the scissors, and the clink of the instruments . . . all are threatening sounds. . . ."[1]

If the baby care unit is out of the mother's field of vision, hearing her baby cry will not reassure her that all is well until she can actually see for herself. Although the immediate ministrations to the baby take just a few minutes, those minutes pass like hours. "Is the baby all right?" "What does she look like?" "Is she *really* okay?" "If she's as healthy as you say she is, why can't I see her?" are questions maternity nurses have probably heard frequently. Placing the baby care unit where the mother can see is so simple, so obvious a solution that many may wonder why it hasn't been done before. In hospitals where it is the standard procedure, congratulations are in order.

As soon as the infant is cared for, she should be brought directly to the mother. Because her arms are otherwise occupied, she will be unable to hold her child. But the nurse will be able to bring the baby close enough so that she can see, kiss, and touch her baby with her face. Just how very, very important this early bodily contact between mother and baby is is discussed in Chapter 15.

Before the baby is taken to the nursery, she should always be presented to the mother. Parents frequently complain that the baby was "whisked" away. If the baby is truly endangered, a brief glance and a kiss on the cheek are preferable to "whisking" the baby away. When the mother has not been able to see her baby, she may visualize problems far worse than the reality. Most cesarean babies are healthy and perfect. Recent studies indicate that even if the baby is severely ill or later succumbs to illness, the grieving process for the parents is less traumatic if they have seen their baby. Almost without exception, the newly delivered cesarean baby can and should be brought to the parents immediately.

When the father is present he will be able to hold the baby and take the child to the mother for stroking, nuzzling, and kissing, and both parents will be able to initiate the bonding process. Touching and bonding which occurs immediately after birth can be more profound than contact which takes place hours or even days later.

While the baby is being cared for and presented to the parents, the obstetrician will begin the final stages of the cesarean procedure. The placenta must be delivered. Usually this large, veined organ comes out intact, and the obstetrician will always make certain that it is fully delivered before suturing. Suturing is the longest part of the cesarean delivery and may require anywhere from 15 to 40 minutes. If the mother is absorbed in her baby she will probably be totally unaware of what is happening—at least until the baby leaves the room. There is no need to hurry with the suturing. The doctor will suture (sew closed) the uterus, the layers of tissue and fiber in the abdominal cavity, and the skin of the abdomen. If the mother has elected to have her tubes tied or her appendix removed, the doctor will do so before closing the abdominal cavity. Women who do not wish to have more children find this an excellent occasion for tubal ligation. The abdomen is already opened, so time, money, and effort are saved and the stress of an additional operation avoided.

The internal stitches will be dissolvable. The skin sutures may be either dissolvable or nonabsorbable. Clamps, rather than stitches, are sometimes used. Nonabsorbable stitches need to be removed on or about the seventh day. If you are still hospitalized, the stitches will be removed before your discharge. Many women are discharged on the fourth or fifth postpartum day, and in such instances, will need to visit the doctor's office or clinic a few days later.

In the space of one hour or so, a baby will have been born by cesarean. The precise teamwork of the doctors and nurses may seem almost nonchalant. It isn't. Years of training, and a great deal of planning have gone into making the procedures appear effortless and routine. For the parents, this is a day so special they will remember it for the rest of their lives. The cesarean baby will benefit from, or be adversely affected both by the quality of the medical, technical, surgical, and anesthetic care the mother receives, and by the concern and support the parents have been accorded. There is a special beauty, a poetry, a spirituality, a closeness that comes from having a baby. For the mother, for the father and for the baby, this has been a birthday! Now is a time to be grateful for the advances of this century, and to rejoice in the safe delivery of a new human being.

CHAPTER 9 BIRTHDAY: A PHOTOESSAY

An hour before the Hills' second cesarean birth, Leslie reads the morning paper while Fred enjoys a continental breakfast provided by the hospital.

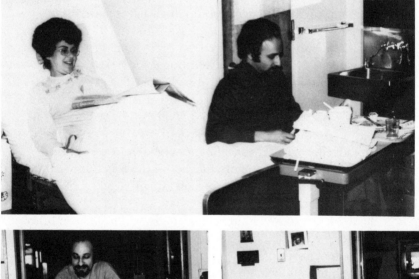

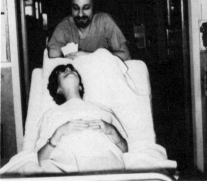

En route to the delivery suite the Hills make bets with each other as to whether two and a half-year-old Heidi will have a brother. The odds are against it, since there hasn't been a boy born into the Hill family in over 30 years.

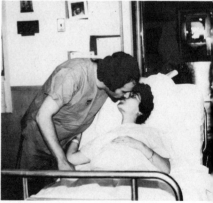

Fred and Leslie exchange kisses before the delivery starts.

Leslie is smiling and confident as the doctors begin.

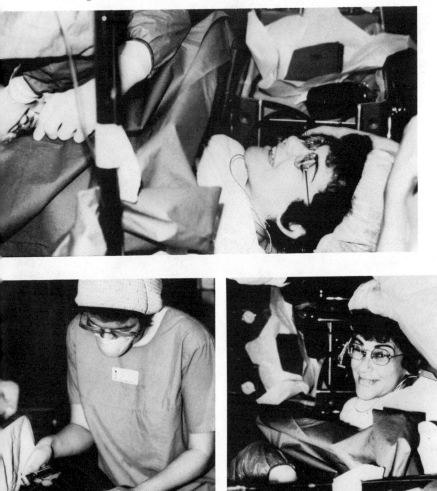

A few minutes later Leslie is relaxed and comfortable again.

A nurse administers oxygen to help Leslie overcome her nausea.

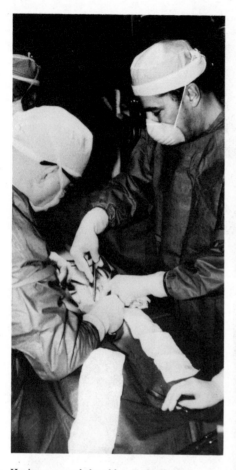

Having removed the old scar, the doctors
reach the layers of tissue beneath the
skin.

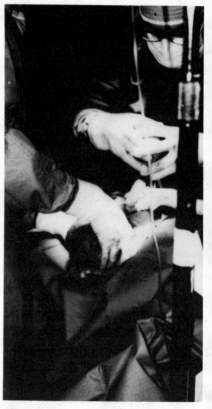

As the assisting physician readies the suction bulb, the baby's head is delivered
by the obstretrician.

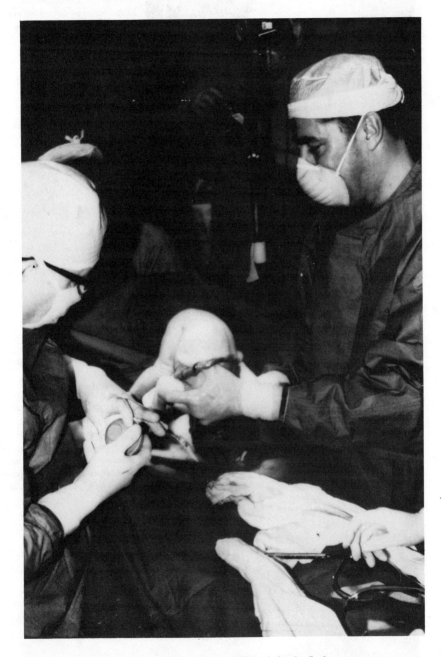

It's a boy! Although most cesarean babies are delivered slowly, Joshua came out rapidly, with the cord wrapped around his body.

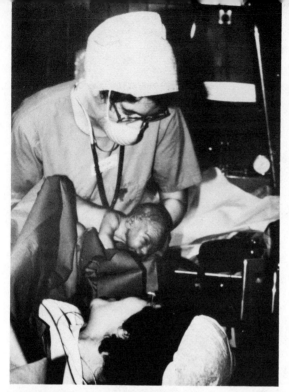

A nurse brings the baby to Leslie for eye-contact before placing him in the receiving bed.

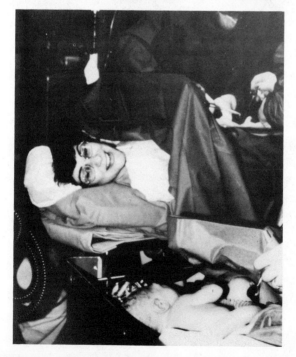

Leslie's attention is completely captured as she sees Joshua pink up within moments of his birth, while the nurse suctions mucus, administers oxygen to ensure an adequate supply, and places places bands on his arm and leg.

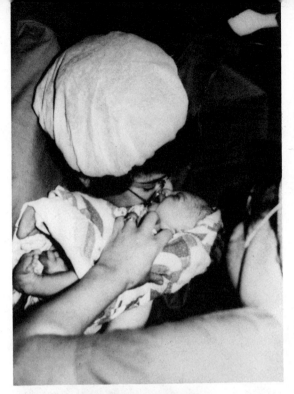

After Joshua has been Apgar-scored at one- and five-minute intervals, he is wrapped in a blanket and brought to Leslie for touching and bonding.

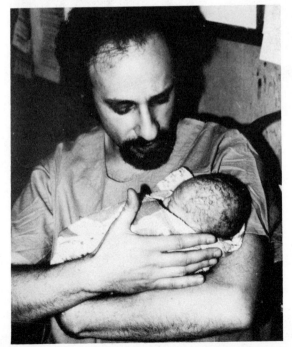

Joshua, age 10 minutes, is held by his father.

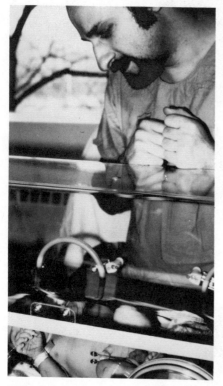

While the delivery continues, Joshua is taken to the special-care nursery for a short observation period.

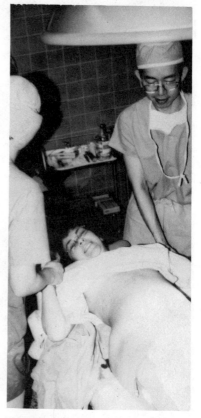

The delivery completed, Leslie is ready to be taken to the recovery room.

Joshua has his first snack while Fred and Leslie call
Heidi and the grandparents from the recovery room.

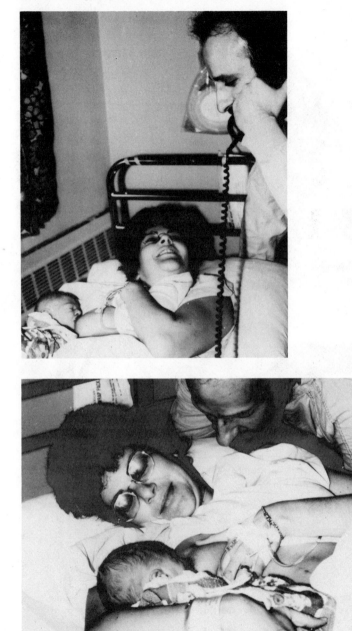

Still in the recovery room, Leslie, Fred, and Joshua spend a few moments
of quiet family togetherness.

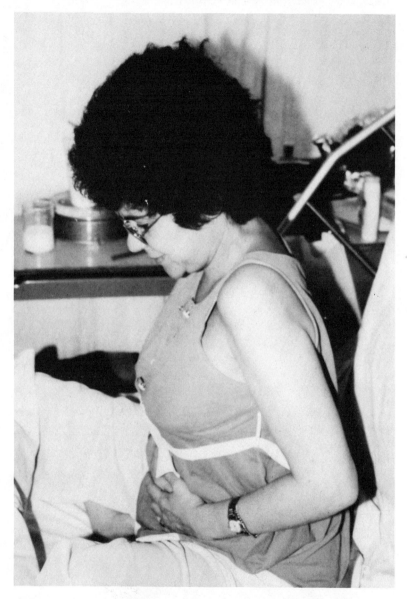

Leslie continues to do the abdominal tightening exercise the next day. Unlike her first cesarean delivery, she has experienced only an hour of mild gas pains this time.

Rooming-in enables Joshua and his parents to become acquainted.

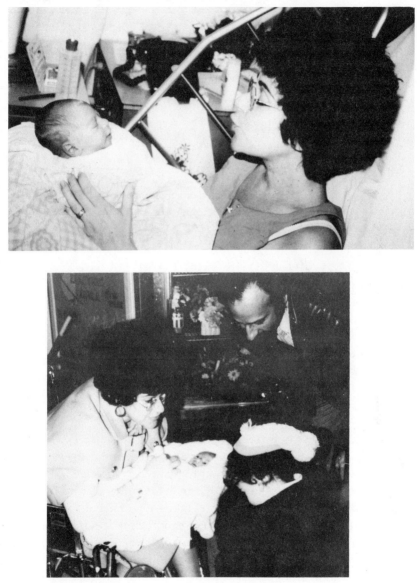

Sister Heidi on being told that Joshua is coming home with the family, experiences temporary uncertainty about having to share Mommy and Daddy with the new baby.

CHAPTER 10 CONTROVERSY: THE FATHER IN THE CESAREAN DELIVERY ROOM

"When I married my wife, I vowed to stay with her for richer for poorer, for better or for worse, in sickness and in health, forever and ever till death do us part.

"Nowhere in our vows did it say that I'd have to leave her if we had a cesarean. I didn't vow to leave her just when we needed each other most."

*D*OES THE FATHER have a right to witness the birth of his baby and to support and comfort his wife when the method of delivery is by cesarean? Is it his right, or a privilege to be extended to a certain few under special circumstances? Is the father who observes a cesarean birth more or less likely to sue the doctor for malpractice? Won't he be a nuisance at best, and a real problem if he faints or becomes sick to his stomach? Isn't he going to get in the way? Why, indeed, should he be there at all? And who would be "crazy" enough to want to watch a surgical birth?

To be sure, these questions are ludicrous in those (few) hospitals where fathers are not as yet allowed in the delivery room for vaginal births. Those nonprogressive, restrictive hospitals aside, the fact remains that many couples wish to be together for the birth of their babies and are permitted to do so more often than not—*unless* a cesarean birth is required. The feasibility of fathers in the cesarean delivery room is a question which stirs passionate debate. In some circles, the mere suggestion causes verbal volcanic eruptions and earthquakes.

Some doctors are afraid that allowing fathers to be present

Myth: Is It Ever Either/Or?

The doctor walks slowly over to a father nervously perched on the arm of a sofa in the waiting room. "I'm sorry," he says to the anxious young man, "You'll have to decide whose life you want to save. Things are really bad. It's got to be either your baby or your wife."

The scene is straight out of a melodrama. It belongs on the shelf beside soap operas (where no woman has ever *had a "good" pregnancy, where babies are born "premature" after 14 months of gestation, and where women have been known to conceive two years after a hysterectomy), next to movies so bad that they are not even run on the late-late-late show. In these movies, the doctor is always male, and portrayed as just slightly higher than the angels. Everyone bows and scrapes to this man, which is understandable, in view of the fact that he has single-handedly cured (and without sleep for at least six months) entire continents from the heartbreak of a particularly virulent strain of psoriasis, while battling creatures from another planet. The situation of an "either/or" decision is not encountered outside the realm of the above-mentioned soaps and soppy movies. Yet it is another myth which persists to this day. If things were really as bad as "all that," the doctor would not have time to come out and ask the father which one he wanted to "save"; he would be too busy in the delivery room for conversation. The heroics have been taken out of childbirth—even childbirth by cesarean. The operation is now so safe that it is almost certain that the father will never be faced with this situation.*

Certain religions traditionally decree that if there is a choice, it is the life of the mother which must be sacrificed in an effort to save and christen the baby. Perhaps this is the origin of the myth. Every effort will be made to save both *the mother and baby. No father should ever be part of the scene above.*

for cesarean births will result in a greater number of malpractice suits. To date there have been no comparative studies made with regard to the incidence of malpractice suits in cesarean deliveries with and without fathers present. However, it is reasonable to speculate that the couple who wish to be together for the birth, and who can see that everything possible is being done for the mother and baby, is the couple who is least likely to bring suit against the doctor. It is also possible that the quality of obstetrical care increases when the father is present.

Time magazine recently carried an article entitled "Malpractice: Rx for a Crisis" which stated:

> Patients rarely sue their family physicians who often make up in compassion and concern what they lack in technical skills. But few feel reluctant to sue an aloof and unfamiliar specialist who seems to take their respect for granted and often submits a sizeable bill as well . . .
>
> Studies have shown that the patient who is treated with compassion is likely to feel that whatever the result, the doctor has done his best. It is the patient who feels himself slighted—in either medical or human terms—who expresses his dissatisfaction by a lawsuit.[1]

One way of assuring a better rapport between the obstetrician and the family is to have the father attend prenatal visits—even if that father is the only male in the waiting room.

Other influential factors in the debate over fathers witnessing cesarean births are tradition ("We just never allowed that before"), hospital policy ("Thou shalt have no fathers in the cesarean section room"), and bias or insecurity on the part of the obstetrician ("I don't want any darned fathers in there looking over my shoulder").

Who would want to watch a baby being delivered by cesarean? Is there a lunatic fringe of fathers out there who crave the chance to see an operation? Do these men want to "peek over the doctor's shoulder" so that they can see how it is done and perform the next cesarean at home on the kitchen table? Do they want only to criticize the doctor's technique?

Although the above paragraph may seem flippant, it is meant seriously, and in the spirit of satire, not sarcasm. One nurse, who wrote on behalf of a doctor, queried, "Is it just certain doctors [in your area] who are performing sections around fathers, or is it more dependent on the situation?" Perhaps it is semantic hairsplitting, but the phrase "*around fathers*" seems to miss the point of why the father is there. The implication is that the father will get in the way, that the obstetrician must step over the father to reach the uterus. The father sits or stands at the head of the delivery table, beside the mother's head, where he can reassure and support her. The father is not there to "see an operation" as such but rather to be with his wife and share with her their baby's birth. The important thing to remember is that the father is just that: a father, a new parent who wishes to be a part of this very special moment in the family's life.

Dr. T. Berry Brazelton wrote, in response to my letter to him:

I personally would like to involve fathers in any phase of or any kind of delivery—for their sakes and for their wives' and babies' future, for I feel that the more involved they are around delivery the more they can be counted on for involvement in the future of the family. But a cesarean is an operative procedure and stressful for the patient, father and doctor. If the latter is under extra stress because of the father's presence, it may be less than optimal for the mother and baby. Of course I would feel that the goal would be to work toward father participation and support in all phases of such an important life's step. I feel this in all aspects of illness and medicine, as well, but even more about a positive step like delivering a baby.[2]

Dr. Brazelton was not asked to nor did he address the question of possible stress on the obstetrician from having medical students present. One mother voiced an opinion shared by other parents, "I told my doctor that if my husband couldn't be there, neither could any student doctors or nurses. I didn't want to be used as a case history if my husband was not permitted to see our baby being born."

Dr. J. Robert McTammany, Chief of Obstetrics at Community General Hospital in Reading, Pennsylvania, who has permitted fathers to be present for cesarean deliveries for several years, has this to say,

It is a pleasure to describe our experiences with family-centered cesarean births. For about two years now we have encouraged fathers to come into the operating room for cesarean births and the program has been an unqualified success. This has been done at Community General Hospital in Reading, Pennsylvania, whose executive committee minutes show, "while non-medical persons are not allowed in the operating rooms of this hospital, it is recognized that a cesarean section is primarily the birth of an infant, and secondarily, a surgical operation, so fathers may be present at cesarean births." We have done between 50 and 100 such births now and have absolutely no reason to regret it or modify the practice in the future.

In most cases, they are primary sections. We indoctrinate the couple as time permits prior to the surgery. If we have to do the delivery hastily (for example, because of fetal distress) we talk with the couple afterwards in more detail. In repeat sections, there is more time for preparation and our CEA [Childbirth Education Association] C-section group is working on a training course for repeat cesarean couples. We have the father present in the room for the induction of anesthesia—usually spinal. He sits off to the side of the room while everything gets going and then sits by his wife's left shoulder during the operation where he can hold her hand and comfort her. (If we have to use general anesthesia, I permit the father to be present anyway, since telling her about the birth and what their baby looked like is of immense value to her). He is told that he may stand up and watch as much or as little of the operation as he likes, and that he may take snapshots if he wishes. When the baby is born it is handed to the waiting delivery room nurse who does what is necessary to the child, and as soon as practicable, wraps the baby in a blanket and gives it to the father who then cuddles the child close and takes it to his wife to see. The three of them spend five or ten minutes together sharing, and the baby is then taken to the nursery for weighing, banding, footprinting, eye-treatment, etc. The father is told he can either go to the nursery with the baby and make phone calls, or stay with his wife for the remainder of the operation and go with her to the recovery room. Most of them stay. Later on they get the baby's weight and make phone calls.

We haven't tried nursing [breastfeeding] in the operating room yet, but often try it several hours later when the mother is back in her bed and recovered from the anesthesia. Many of the mothers go home on their third post-operative day and they do beautifully.

It is all so simple and so right. Many couples just accept it as the natural thing to do and don't understand what an unusual opportunity they have had. All are very impressed with the o.r. [operating room] routine and teamwork. In cases where there are problems—with the mother or baby—the father lends his support and sees for himself all of our efforts on behalf of the person in trouble. They feel a tremendous appreciation—almost unworthiness—for all that is done.

The same joy and excitement we have in the delivery room is, in this way, experienced in the operating room. It seems even a little more intense because there are more participants and there is great release when the outcome is successful.

Other doctors in the area are becoming enthusiastic about doing this and just recently Reading's largest hospital began to let fathers in. Some of them are reluctant to do it however, fearing lawsuits or feeling insecure. The only lawsuit I ever had was in a case where the father did not want to come in. . . . I feel if anything, it lessens the likelihood of lawsuits.[3]

Being the father of a baby who decides to come into the world through an abdominal incision rather than the birth canal may create special problems. The cesarean father usually has no glowing tales of how beautifully labor progressed with his wife's efforts and his coaching and support. He will be unable to reflect on the feelings of exultation and pride that he experienced as the baby's head, and then body emerged. There will seldom be lovely pictures for the family album to be cherished, admired, and passed on to the child. The cesarean couple will be unable to reminisce about the time of joy and happiness they shared as the baby is born *unless* the couple have an understanding doctor and a supportive hospital policy.

Usually, while the mother is in the cesarean delivery room, the father is helpless, alone, and ignored. He may be alternately apprehensive about the safety and well-being of the mother and baby, and eager for the long-awaited birth of his child. He is not allowed to support his wife as he wants, as he thinks he should, if only he were given the opportunity. In fact, the father may be unable to see either the mother or the baby until hours after the delivery, thereby missing the chance to reassure himself and the baby's mother that all is well. If the father must wait in the lobby or fathers' room, it is important that the hospital staff keep him informed.

A woman from Illinois reports, "I guess my husband was rather worried. They took me to the operating room at 10:50

and he never heard anything until around 1:30. They didn't start surgery right away, and then after the baby was born they did a complete check on the baby before they gave me a tubal. My first emergency section took twenty minutes, and this one over two hours. They said in a routine section they just don't worry about time, and forget sometimes to let the father know. . . ." Her letter highlights the necessity of keeping fathers informed and reassured.

What can be done to make it possible for willing fathers to share their babies' birth? The most valuable aid to changing current policies and practices is *consumer pressure.* Letters to hospital administrators, executive boards, doctors—even letters to the editors of local newspapers may help to gain support from hospitals and doctors. The best (and first—as well as nicest) way to approach the subject is to have a talk with your doctor and the administrator of the hospital. You should not expect this first meeting to result in instant total policy changes. An amiable presentation of your case will help to open the door. Sometimes the greatest opposition comes from the anesthesia department. This opposition is somewhat understandable, in view of the fact that the anesthesiologist has the most vital job of anyone in the delivery room (keeping the mother comfortable and alive), and therefore, their insurance premiums are often the highest of any medical specialty. Anesthesiologists have (potentially) the most to lose should a parent file suit and win.

One of the most frustrating problems the parents may encounter is that of "corporate structure." In other words, their personal obstetrician may be quite willing to allow them to be together, but permission from other departments or the administrative office may be unattainable. It is also fairly common to find that permission is granted by one department or individual, but that colleagues refuse to go along. One department may say, "Sure, we think it's a great idea, but the other department won't grant permission." When the other department is contacted, the reply may be, "Yes, we think it's a good idea but the people in administration don't want to do it." Passing the buck isn't always intentional, but it is frustrating.

There may be hospitals in the United States and Canada where fathers were never refused permission to be present for cesarean births. However, until fairly recently, there were probably few couples who even bothered to ask, assuming that their request would be considered outlandish or bizarre. There are other hospitals, such as Boston Hospital for Women, Lying-In Division, and Community General Hospital in Reading, Pennsylvania, where the policy of allowing fathers to be present has been in effect for several years. Interestingly enough, changes in one hospital's policy often cause changes in other, nearby hospitals. Whether this phenomenon is due to competition among hospitals for patients, or to a true concern for their patients' welfare is subject to speculation. In the cases of Boston (where at least seven or eight hospitals in the metropolitan area now permit fathers to be present), and Reading, Pennsylvania (where two out of three hospitals permit fathers in attendance) the change in policy at one hospital *did* indeed have an effect on other area hospitals.

If you live in an area where there is a choice of hospitals, and you elect to change obstetricians and hospitals so that you can be together, be sure to write to your former doctor and hospital administrators telling them *why* you have made the switch. The former obstetrician may assume that you have simply moved away. And hospitals, which often vie for patients, may be more willing to change their policies if they think not doing so will mean an economic loss. Years ago, when the subject of having fathers present for vaginal deliveries was a controversial issue, many doctors changed their attitudes, and hospitals their policies, when it was discovered that patients were going to other hospitals to have their babies. If cesarean parents exert this same economic impact, it may lead to more hospitals granting permission for fathers to attend cesarean deliveries.

Occasionally, even when permission cannot be granted

generally to all parents, individual exceptions can sometimes be made. For example, if the obstetrician is aware that the mother-to-be is especially apprehensive, arrangements can sometimes be made to have the father present. Hospitals which use the regular operating rooms for cesarean deliveries (because they do not have a special cesarean delivery room within the maternity suite) often have the most difficulty changing their policies. A C/SEC, Inc., newsletter tells how one couple was able to overcome this situation by persuading the hospital to have the cesarean take place in a regular delivery room, rather than an o.r. Hospitals which have rigid policies, not subject to change in the near future, may also arrange for fathers to stand in the open doorway just outside the cesarean delivery room. Although he will be unable to hold the mother's hand and support her, he *will* be able to hear his baby's first cries, and to see his baby as soon as it is delivered. This alternative is *not* preferable to having him at his wife's side if that is where he and she want him to be. But it is more reassuring and positive for the couple than making the father wait in a room far away, unable to hear or see any of the baby's birth.

The ecstasy of birth can be heightened when the father is present, and fathers in the cesarean delivery room may make the difference between a successful *surgical* procedure (from a medical standpoint), and a happy, meaningful occasion for the parents and their baby. If the father cannot be present, the hospital staff must act as the "significant other(s)" in his stead.

Judith Gundersen, R.N., and Coordinator of Parent Education at Boston Hospital for Women gives a well-rounded, practical guide for other hospitals wishing to implement policy changes. As one of the first hospitals in the country to implement change, the experience of Boston Hospital for Women may help to guide others:

The hospital has allowed fathers to be present for cesarean childbirths for approximately three years and has had over 300 couples participate thus far. Originally because some members of the medical staff objected to the routine presence of fathers at cesarean births, the obstetrician was required to act as the patient's "advocate" by requesting permission from the Chief of Staff. Generally, if the doctor requested it, permission was given by Dr. Kenneth Ryan, Chief of Staff.

In a revised issue of "Prerequisites for Presence in Labor and Delivery" dated 7/23/75, the current procedure is listed: "The father (surrogate) may be present during Cesarian Section if prior approval has been obtained from the Obstetrician, the Anesthesiologist, and the Charge Nurse." The obstetricians are still also using the formal written procedure as it has been found to insure excellent inter-departmental communications (nursing gets a copy, for instance) and statistical accuracy.

I should also note that fathers are not allowed if the patient is asleep since one of his prime purposes is not needed . . . to provide support for the mother (although it was recently noted that mothers who are asleep may need that reassurance and verification that it *is* their baby since they did not witness its birth . . . witnessing the birth assists the maternal-infant bonding process. See recent writings of Marshall Klaus, M.D., of Cleveland).

Therefore, fathers are usually present for scheduled cesareans, although their presence at unscheduled cesareans is not precluded by the policy, most obstetricians do not encourage it. In our prepared childbirth classes, therefore, we are encouraging couples to discuss the possibility of unscheduled cesarean births and asking their obstetricians to allow the father's presence should one occur. I should clarify that many will allow fathers for unscheduled cesareans (failure to progress, CPD, etc.) as opposed to emergency/unscheduled cesareans (prolapsed cord, bleeding, etc.), for which fathers have not yet been allowed.

While I have not been personally acquainted with all of the couples, I have had contact with many and am always happy anew to share their joy—a joy in sharing birth; not separated and relegated to being a "section" . . . as one couple noted (prior to this policy's inception), "It's as though having a baby is a side effect when you deliver by cesarean."

I am happy to tell you that the original questions and objections raised by members of the nursing, medical and/or administrative staffs have not seemed to materialize (it is interesting that these are areas of concern which echo similarly to those raised re: fathers in the vaginal delivery room):

Father as a contaminant . . . properly suited, booted, capped and masked, he appears to be no more or less a contaminant than any other person in the room.

Father is in the way . . . (Ask any mother about that!) Seriously, any small amount of room he occupies is more than compensated for by the reassurance, comfort and support he provides. In reality, he does not move about the room, but sits at the right or left shoulder on a stool.

In a recent cesarean, when Milton Alper, Chief of the Anesthesia Department had completed his ministrations to the patient prior to the commencement of surgery he asked, "Is there anything else I can get you?" she replied, "All I need is my husband."

Father will be ill, faint, etc. . . . . It has been our observation (as with vaginal births) that the father is so engrossed in his role as supporter, with the progression of the birth, and later with holding the newborn, that his focus of attention is directed away from himself. Any father who has ever experienced any weak-kneed feelings says it occurs *after* the event is over when he has had time to ponder the enormity of the event witnessed. Properly prepared in a course for cesarean childbirth, the father's understanding and awareness of the sequence of events and the reasons why certain procedures are done reassures any concerns he may originally have.

Being sued . . . I believe there is probably less chance of questions arising involving malpractice if any anxious and interested father is allowed to be in the operating room when a cesarean birth is performed. As a lawyer-husband observed, "I was so impressed with the care given my wife and child, the concern rendered, and the reasons for each procedure being done. Everyone was certainly functioning at a very high level of expertise." This observation is repeated to us frequently.

I should add that although the father's presence is primarily for support of the mother, and to share together the moment of birth (but not necessarily to watch the birth as he is sitting behind the ether screen), recently several fathers have asked for, and received permission to, witness the actual birth, thus being the first to tell the mother the sex of their child—no need to tell you all the feeling and meaning engendered by this.

I certainly do not mean to merely wax eloquent about this subject, because, of course, we are talking about major surgery. Procedures and precautions must be established, and each hospital must work out its own requirements. All of this does involve a certain measure of time and input from various departments, but two very definite benefits (to us) have already been demonstrated repeatedly: first, in explaining procedures more thoroughly, I believe we are becoming better practitioners (from nurses, doctors, anesthesiologists, technicians). We see the need for this preparation of patients in other aspects of our jobs, not just the cesarean couple sharing the birth of their child. I also believe it tends to make us relate better to patients as people with needs, not just as patients.

Secondly, the time spent is definitely not wasted time; it is, in fact, reaping significant rewards. Because the couple is so prepared, they function more intelligently and cooperatively in their recovery and learning processes with the newborn. And although this may be nearly impossible to document, there are simply too many couples (who have prepared for and shared the cesarean birth) having quicker and more positive recoveries. It seems that in returning the event of birth (not just surgery) to the couple, we are returning all the positive feelings that birth encompasses: positive self-image; pride of accomplishment in a procreative ability; and a heightened awareness of the marital relationship.

Fathers, too, do not hesitate to acknowledge the benefits to themselves. Just this past week, a "repeat" father told his instructor, "We now have two children, but only now do I feel we have given birth." He noted that he couldn't help but be more supportive, more understanding, more physically helpful with chores, the new baby, etc.

Comments like the above are repeated again and again, and I encourage your efforts to bring family-centered cesarean births to your hospital. I have shared the sense of awe James Stanton, our Director, has felt talking with couples from Michigan and Pennsylvania who have flown to Boston to have their babies here as their hospitals would not allow the father to be present for the cesarean birth! We are certainly *not* encouraging couples to do this, and are actively engaged in a letter-writing campaign when requested to do so to encourage more hospitals to allow cesarean births to be shared.[4]

Yes, cesarean fathers *do* have a right to be present for their babies' births. Sadly, it may take several years before all hospitals make this much-needed, much-demanded policy change, but more and more hospitals have recently enacted changes. It is an idea whose time has come. It will take time, effort, and the cooperation of parents, doctors, and hospital administrators. And, it is worth it. Good luck.

CHAPTER 11 THE RECOVERY ROOM:
A GOOD BEGINNING

*T*HE AMOUNT OF TIME the new mother spends in the recovery room is, on the average, about three hours. It will be necessary to remain longer if there are special problems. The recovery room staff is experienced in caring for the postpartum patient, and if the maternity floor is very busy, the mother may be kept in the recovery room for longer than three hours to ensure careful, constant checking of her condition.

Some hospitals do not have an obstetrical recovery room. Newly delivered cesarean mothers may be kept in the corridor of the labor and delivery area, or in an empty labor room, or in the regular surgical recovery room, or they may be taken immediately back to their rooms on the maternity floor. If the mother has had general anesthesia, she may remember very little of this period regardless of where it takes place. Once the mother has begun to awaken and it has been ascertained that her condition is stable, she will be returned to her room. Additional medications may keep her fairly groggy for at least another eight hours after the baby is born.

If the couple have had to be separated for the baby's birth, it is often possible (and always preferable) to be reunited with the baby's father in the recovery room. (If your hospital does not have a separate maternity recovery room, some of the procedures and suggestions of this chapter may be inapplicable.) The recovery room nurses usually try to maintain a low profile for at least the first few minutes after the mother and father are together again, so that the parents can love and comfort one another, and privately rejoice in the birth of their baby. The couple may have been separated for as little as one hour, but those 60 minutes have been more significant than any other hour in their lives.

A telephone may be available in the recovery room so that the new mother and father can announce the baby's birth to relatives. The baby's father or a recovery room nurse should dial long-distance numbers. It is too draining for the new mother to have to go through the rigamarole of charging numbers to her room or home phone, calling person-to-person, collect, etc.

Announcing the birth within minutes after delivery is exciting to the proud parents, grandparents, and older children. Talking to Mommy will reassure older children, and make them feel a part of the new baby's arrival. However, some children react nonchalantly to the announcement—and this seeming lack of interest surprises and dismays some parents. It is not cause for concern or disappointment. Older children may have been prepared well in advance for the arrival of their new little sister or brother, but until they can actually see and touch the baby for themselves, they may not fully comprehend its significance. Often they say, "Oh, really?" and then launch into an account of what they have been doing.

In the excitement and stress of giving birth, many women will become sweaty or clammy, and among the first things that will take place in the recovery room is that the mother will be given a bed bath, and helped to change into a clean hospital gown. This bath can be soothing and welcome—especially if it is done gently. A mouthwash or toothbrush may be offered. Vital signs (temperature, pulse, and blood pressure) will be taken every 15 minutes or more often if necessary. The amount, consistency, and color of the vaginal discharge will be checked frequently. This flow will last from two to six weeks. The recovery room nurse will also check the incision and the height of the top of the uterus. This is determined by pressing on the abdomen, but sometimes the abdomen is so tender that even the most gentle pressure is excruciatingly painful. If you think the nurse is exerting too much pressure, ask her to be gentler. These examinations take just a few seconds, but they are done frequently and are very important. It takes about six weeks for the uterus to return to its normal, nonpregnant size, but there will be a dramatic, rapid shrinking immediately after delivery. A uterus that contracts surely and rapidly is a uterus that is less likely to become infected or to hemorrhage.

To help stimulate contraction of the uterus, pitocin may be added to the intravenous solution. Pitocin (sometimes called "pit") is the same substance that is used to stimulate or induce labor. As the uterus contracts of its own accord, and/or with the help of pitocin, the mother may experience contractions like those of labor. The intensity of these contractions varies from woman to woman, and from one pregnancy to another. Should the contractions become painful at any time, or should you feel as though you are having one continuous, uninter-rupted contraction, be sure to tell the nurse. Mild cramping at intervals is to be expected. Continual pain is not. The pito-cin may be flowing too rapidly from the i.v. The nurse will be able to slow down the i.v. or discontinue the pitocin altogether (with your doctor's permission) or give additional pain medi-cation if necessary. A few mild cramps can be managed with pain medication and/or slow, controlled relaxation breathing. It is thought that postpartum contractions may be more intense with second and subsequent pregnancies, although the reasons are still the subject of medical study. The cesarean mother should remember that she has had a baby, and that her body must make adjustments to compensate for the swift change from mother-to-be to mother-in-fact. (Incidentally, the pitocin may be continued for at least a few hours after the mother has been returned to her room on the postpartum floor, so the problem of intense after-birth contractions, if it is to occur, may not surface until then.)

Soon after she has been taken to the recovery room, the mother's legs will regain sensation if she has had spinal anesthesia. Sometimes the legs begin to tingle or feel the way legs do when they have fallen asleep. The sensation usually begins at the toes and progresses upwards. The nurse will ask the mother to move her legs. At first, her brain may send the command, but receive no response. Gradually motor control will return. This regaining of sensation has been described by different mothers as being "weird," "prickly," and "oddly uncomfortable"—but never painful.

In the recovery room, one or more injections may be given to alleviate pain. These may make the mother sleepy, groggy, or drowsy. At this time, the excitement of the day's events combined with the physical strains of the cesarean delivery may make the mother feel "spaced out" or "out of it completely." Some mothers are so happy and high that sleep is out of the question. They chat with the baby's father and talk the nurses' ears off. The mother who does feel sleepy is encouraged to give in to that feeling. If the father is there, he will certainly understand that this rest is beneficial.

The amount of discomfort experienced in the recovery room (and during the remainder of the hospital stay) varies from woman to woman, and even from delivery to delivery. Some mothers feel little or no discomfort, while others report that they were totally miserable and in severe pain. How much pain you experience should *not* be considered a negative reflection on your coping abilities. If at any time you feel uncomfortable or unable to cope effectively, inform the nurses immediately. Most obstetricians make only brief rounds, so it is the nurses on whom you must depend. They, in turn, will communicate any special problems requiring immediate attention to your obstetrician.

As a general rule throughout the hospital stay, it is a good idea to take pain medication before discomfort becomes severe. This way the medication will work more effectively and sooner. Playing "Superwoman" or trying to "tough it out" without any medication at all is not necessary, nor even especially helpful. You have had a baby and an operation. A cesarean delivery is not an endurance test. Feeling uncomfortable does not mean that you are a "weakling" or a "failure." Knowing what to expect and how to cope effectively with any situation will help to make your recuperative period easier.

Headaches, as the direct result of anesthesia, will occur within a few hours or days of delivery *if* they are to happen at all. (Anesthesia will not be the cause of headaches which occur months or years after delivery.) You may experience shoulder pain—a result of air having collected under the diaphragm as a result of surgery. Tell the doctor or nurse if either headache or shoulder pain, or both, happen. They are not major problems, but can be aggravating especially in conjunction with the other physical debilities which may occur as the result of just having delivered a baby by cesarean. Because of new techniques headaches from anesthesia are less frequent nowadays.

Both the bladder catheter and the i.v. (intravenous) will remain in place. How soon either or both are removed depends on the doctor's orders and the mother's condition. Some doctors prefer to have them kept in place for a day or two.

Equally important as the physical care the mother receives in the recovery room is the fulfillment of her need to begin the "mothering" processes. For healthy, normal mothering patterns to flourish and grow, the mother and her baby must be reunited as soon as possible. While the anesthesia is still partially in effect, the mother should be quite comfortable physically. Coupled with the elation of giving birth, the first hour or two in the recovery room is a superb time for mother and father to become acquainted with their baby, and for the mother to initiate breastfeeding. Even if she does not breastfeed, early, close physical contact will promote the maternal-infant bonding processes, and reassure mother, father, and baby. (See chapter 15.)

What will make the mother most happy in the recovery room is to have her baby brought to her there. She may have been able to kiss and touch her new baby in the delivery room, but holding her baby in her arms is an experience without equal. Unless the baby is truly endangered and cannot be taken from the special care nursery, both mother and baby will benefit from this early, close contact. The baby will be reassured by her mother's heartbeat, a sound which has been familiar to her during the entire gestation process. The mother will be able to examine closely her baby and to see for herself that the child is well. No matter what anyone else tells her about her baby's perfection nothing can replace her own inspection.

The mother will need help holding and feeding her baby. The nurse or baby's father can make the mother comfortable by helping her to turn on her side, by propping pillows under her back, by adjusting the bed for comfort, and by helping her to loosen her hospital gown so that her baby can have skin-to-skin contact and access to her mother's breast. The baby's father may lift the child from her crib and place the infant in the mother's arms. This contact will help to promote his sense of closeness to the baby.

Newborn babies are often "barracudas" and take to sucking with vigor. Snuggling together, with the nurse and baby's father beside her to lend the assurance new mothers need (they need to know that they are doing a good job of caring for their babies) will promote the mother's sense of security. This reinforcement of her caretaking abilities is especially important if, instead of a "go-getter" or "barracuda," the baby is sleepy and won't nurse right away.

When the mother has finished nursing on one breast, the baby's father can bubble the baby, place her in her crib, and then rearrange the pillows and help the mother turn onto her other side for feeding. There should always be a pillow on the

mother's lap to splint the incision and take the pressure of
the baby's body off this very tender area.

The benefits of nursing the baby within a short time after
birth are numerous and vital. They include mother-baby skin
contact, the reassurance to the baby of the mother's heartbeat,
the immunities provided by the colostrum (the first milk
secreted), baby-father contact and bonding, baby-mother
bonding, even a new mother-father bonding, face-to-face
contact and tactile stimulation of the infant; and the flow of
love which only the parents can give, however "inexpert"
they may feel initially. Some newborns have trouble maintaining a stable body temperature. Being held in the mother's
arms may help. The warmth of a mother's body is the best
baby-warmer unit ever devised. The parents may be concerned
at first that they won't know how to hold the baby properly,
that they will not know what to do for or with her. Even
if the baby is a 10-pounder, she will look so helpless, so tiny,
so fragile. She isn't as delicate as she looks.

The mother will also need coddling and care right after
birth. She may be exhausted as the result of having had a
cesarean, and then from holding her baby. While the baby is
with her, she may be so enthralled and ecstatic that she forgets
about herself. When the baby is taken back to the nursery,
the mother may welcome the opportunity to fall blissfully
asleep. The first contact in the recovery room between mother
and baby need not be more than a few minutes—but it is an
important time.

If the baby cannot be brought to the mother in the recovery
room (either because of rigid, old-fashioned hospital policy,
or because the baby *must* remain in the special care nursery
where her condition can be monitored, the amount of oxygen
she receives regulated, and the temperature and humidity
controlled), the baby's father or surrogate (a special friend or
relative who has received permission to take his place) may
wish to take Polaroid pictures of the baby at frequent intervals
to show to the mother. Good communications between the

nursery staff and the recovery room nurses is essential at all times—but particularly if inflexible hospital policy dictates that the mother cannot have anyone with her in the recovery room. Even when the baby's father is with the mother, and the baby is to be brought to her, there is usually a short observation period varying from a few minutes to a few hours, depending on hospital policy, the availability of a pediatrician or special nurse to give the go-ahead, and/or the baby's temperature. Usually there is a drop in the baby's temperature immediately after birth. Before the baby can be brought to the mother, her temperature must rise to normal and remain stable. During this time, the mother may ask and re-ask for frequent reports on the baby's condition. The reporter may become a bit exasperated, but until the mother can see for herself, this constant reiteration is vitally important to her.

Some hospitals have Polaroid cameras on the maternity floor for use by parents. It is better to bring your own (and lots of film) since not all hospitals have cameras. These photographs can bring immediate reassurance to the mother and will later be treasured by the parents—even if they are a little disappointed at first at the appearance of their baby. Newborns are often wrinkly, scrunched up, and less than glamorous. Bringing your own instant camera will also enable you to take lots of pictures for the grandparents and older children. The new mother who cannot have her baby for hours (or, in a few cases, days) will want to have pictures taken frequently because the newborn baby changes rapidly—sometimes even from one hour to the next.

ABDOMINAL TIGHTENING EXERCISE TO REDUCE GAS DISCOMFORT

Although gas pains do not usually occur until several days after delivery, one hour after the baby's birth is the time to begin using this technique to help reduce (and in some cases, eliminate) what many mothers call "the *worst* aspect of having a cesarean"—gas. After a cesarean, the condition is *never* "only gas." It is GAS and it can hurt!

Gas forms because the intestines have temporarily stopped working efficiently due to the fact that (1) the mother has had anesthesia and a host of other medications; (2) the intestines have been exposed to air and handled during the operation; and (3) the mother is unable to move about freely as is necessary to help stimulate normal intestinal action. Not every cesarean mother gets a painful bout of gas. For those who do, the suffering it produces varies from mild to severe. For maximum effect, begin this abdominal tightening exercise within one hour after delivery, and do it four or five times an hour *every* hour that you are awake for at least five days. Although this technique can be used by anyone who has undergone abdominal surgery, an added bonus for the cesarean mother is that it will make it easier for her to move about comfortably and to care for her baby the first few postpartum days. Here is the exercise recommended by Valmai Elkins, Registered Physical Therapist of Montreal.

First, place both hands over your incision to form a splint. If you like, place a small pillow directly over your abdomen for further support, and then join both hands together on top of the pillow, just over the incision. Take a deep "welcoming" breath in and then let it all out. Take another deep breath and hold it to the slow count of 5. Holding to the count of 10 is better if you can manage it but don't push yourself too hard, at least the first few times you try. When you have finished counting, let the breath out, and take a final deep "parting" breath in and let it out.

The hospital where you deliver may already use this technique, and one of the recovery room nurses may remind you to begin abdominal tightening as a matter of postoperative routine. If not, ask your husband to put this on his checklist of things to do. The first few times you try this technique it may be uncomfortable. It becomes easier each time. Also, you

may be afraid to do it for fear the incision may come apart.
That won't happen. Abdominal tightening is imperative to
help make your recovery smoother and more comfortable.

A GOOD BEGINNING

In the recovery room you may feel a combination of physical
sensations, euphoria, triumph, jubilance, fatigue, and relief.
A good recovery room experience, like a good delivery, will
be a positive beginning for you as a family. Uniting parents
and baby in the recovery room is a way of making the cesarean
delivery a family-centered event, and will see you off to a good
relationship with your baby, and your baby with you.

The long wait is over. The baby is healthy, beautiful, and
yours for keeps. Hallelujah! Now it is time to rejoice, relax,
and begin to recover.

CHAPTER 12 THE POSTPARTUM
HOSPITAL STAY

*T*O PARAPHRASE Reeva Rubin, professor and director of the Graduate Program in Maternity Nursing at the University of Pittsburgh, it's pretty hard to feel maternal when your mouth tastes like last week's garbage, and your back feels like a twisted lead pipe. Cesarean mothers are handicapped by a lack of mobility and by physical discomfort which sometimes makes it difficult for them to establish their roles as caretaker and nurturer in the first few days and weeks after birth. The cesarean mother needs rest, relaxation, and support. In a word: she, too, needs coddling.

The hospital stay will be about five days. Some women are released after two or three days, most stay five, and a few require a week or more. Try not to be in a hurry to get home. An extra day or two in the hospital (especially if there is an older child or children at home, and/or adequate help is not available) may be beneficial.

A very few women breeze through the recovery period. Their incisions cause only minor concern. Nothing bothers them, not their own bodies, nor the needs of the newborn. They are ecstatic. Within a few days of delivery, they are happy and home. Within weeks, they may be doing all the things they normally did before the baby was born and may even tackle some tasks such as wallpapering the baby's room which other mothers cannot do for months.

At the other end of the spectrum are women who, through no fault of their own, have complications. Their incisions may become infected; they may develop a high fever or hemorrhaging may occur; a totally unrelated illness such as the flu or a cold strikes them; or they may suffer a reaction to one of the drugs administered. No matter how positive their attitudes, their bodies are truly debilitated. Complications do *not* usually occur—but they can happen.

There is a tiny group of mothers who, like characters from soap operas, use their birthing experiences as convenient pegs on which to hang *all* their troubles. From the moment they awaken from anesthesia and for years afterward, their "horrible, just *horrible*" operation is a favorite topic. Everything which happens to them from then on is blamed on their "sections." (These women do not give birth by cesarean, they have Sections, with a capital "S".)

The vast majority of cesarean mothers fall somewhere in the middle of the spectrum. They, too, must talk about and relive their experiences. It is natural and healthy. Talking about what happened will enable them to finalize the experience. These women are delighted to be mothers, but their bodies are not as cooperative as their minds. They cannot move freely. Walking, sneezing, laughing, and coughing become "unnatural" and painful. Their bodies need time to repair themselves, and their babies want to snuggle, nurse, and be loved at the same time. What can be done to help smooth over the first few postpartum days? There are steps which the mother, father, and hospital staff can take which will have very positive effects on the way the parents relate to the baby and which will help to transform the "container of pain" into a comfortable, loving mother.

The first 24 hours or so after delivery will probably be fairly hazy. Fatigue, pain medication, and a sense of relief and accomplishment make the new mother very tired. You may remember very little of what happens the first day. Relax and take it easy. Your body will dictate how much or how little you *should* do. You have just given birth and deserve to think only of yourself—for a few hours, at least. If you force yourself too much, you will not make a very cheerful mother when the baby is brought to you. If you want to have full rooming-in, you may prefer to initiate it after you've had a day or two in which to regain your strength.

It is essential to continue the abdominal tightening exercise (see Chapter 11). If you forgot to begin in the recovery room, it is never too late, although maximum benefit may be reduced. Not all hospitals are as yet familiar with this exercise, and you may be asked what you're doing and why.

Both to relieve gas and to speed the recuperative period, it is best to turn as often and as frequently as possible while you are still confined to bed. It is probably going to hurt at first, especially if you have a classical incision. Relaxation breathing techniques will help those first few times you shift your position. It gets easier each time.

Check your position in bed several times a day. As the day progresses, you may end up "scrunched up" at the foot of the bed. Try to remember to keep yourself in a lying down flat or sitting position.

Within 24 hours of delivery, you will take your first trip out of bed. Even if you are feeling on top of the world, the first trip should not be undertaken unless there is a nurse in the room. You will need her help in case you get dizzy or feel faint. Just the effort of sitting up the first time may make you feel dizzy. The baby's father may be present at this time, but other visitors should not be. Getting out of bed and walking to a chair will require a great deal of effort. Also, the effort may possibly cause a sudden, profuse gush of vaginal discharge which you may find embarrassing if there are other people in the room.

The most outstanding sensation every new cesarean mother has as she tries to sit up, swing her legs over the side of the bed, and stand is a pulling or tugging in the area around the incision. In fact, if this is your first cesarean, this feeling may come as an unpleasant shock. You may think your incision is going to split apart and the entire contents of your insides tumble out onto the floor. The incision will not come apart, but it is a feeling experienced by almost every cesarean mother. To compensate for this sensation, which may be experienced as a minor feeling of discomfort, or as a searing pain, you will be inclined to bend from the waist, to stoop, and to do what is called the "cesarean shuffle." Don't. The "cesarean shuffle" is highly discouraged, even though it may take a great deal of effort to stand straight and tall. The incision will heal better and more attractively if you remember to walk like a high-fashion model the first and every time that you walk. How bad it can hurt to stand and walk should not be minimized. It may hurt like the blue blazes. Fortunately, it gets easier each time. The more you move about, the earlier you do so—and the straighter you stand—the sooner you will be able to move gracefully and effortlessly.

The first walk (which some mothers liken to the "incredible journey" in *Pilgrim's Progress*) can be accomplished even if the i.v. and catheter are still in place. It may seem to take forever just to walk from the bed to a chair a few feet away.

What and when you are allowed to eat depends on your doctor's preferences and your condition. The i.v. may be kept running for several days. Through the i.v. you will receive water, glucose or dextrose (sugar), saline (salt), and/or medications. You may be allowed only room-temperature water and juices for days, while another cesarean mother, who delivered the same time you did, may be served dinner that evening. She probably has another doctor. The major reason for conservatism with regard to diet is the belief that limiting the diet may reduce the discomforts of gas and constipation.

Being very, very thirsty after having a baby is not uncommon. Water, regardless of its temperature, is a welcome thirst-quencher. From water, you may progress to broth, juices, and soda (cola, ginger ale, etc.)—although it is advisable to sip

carbonated beverages through a straw after some of the
bubbles have dissipated. Gelatin will probably be the first food
you will be allowed to eat. After all those liquids, the first
few dishes are very tasty, but then you may notice that breakfast, lunch and dinner all bear a disheartening resemblance:
gelatin or custard, clear broth, and tea. That is fine—for a
while. After what seems like an eternity of broth, tea, and gelatin, you may become so hungry that you would do anything
to have some real food. When the nurse walks into your room
carrying still another tray of custard and broth, your reaction
may be to cry or get angry.

Finally, it is demoralizing to be forbidden "real" foods for
a period of days. Cesarean mothers and their obstetricians
are often able to compromise. Herb teas, yogurt, mashed
potatoes, creamed soups and vegetables, roast turkey and
chicken, broiled fish, rice cereal, or farina may be foods which
the doctor will allow. They will satisfy the mother's hunger,
her body's need for nutrition, and concurrently lift her morale
without adding undue strain on her digestive system.

If you really must have something solid to eat, and your
doctor forbids it for longer than you think necessary, you
could cheat. You could sneak a few cookies, a candy bar, or
something forbidden. If you do, you'll suffer for it. Such
foods are certain to cause gas pains and may lead to constipation. Try to be reasonable and intelligent in making a
decision like that.

The subject of adequate, proper nutrition following surgery
is just now being reevaluated by the medical profession. Some
doctors are well acquainted with the intense needs of the postsurgical patient for vitamins, minerals, and trace elements. It
is known that they are greatly depleted during physical
trauma. Some of these elements can be stored in the body and
released into the system gradually. Others must be replenished
daily. If you are concerned about the need for adequate nutrition, you should discuss it with your obstetrician, preferably
during a prenatal visit. If your doctor prefers a truly conserva-

tive diet, you may request vitamin tablets to give a much-needed boost during those first few days when you are restricted as to what you may eat and drink.

Pain medication will be offered for at least two or three days and probably longer. At first, it will be given as an injection and later as pills. It is true that some of this medication will go through the mother's milk and into the baby. The amount passed on to the baby is minimal, and the mother may find it difficult indeed to be really "maternal" if she is in pain. Pain may vary from mild discomfort to a temporarily excruciating sensation. There are times when you will want to take the medication offered—and may even find it difficult to wait for the next dose. At other times, your need may not be as great. You'll discover how often you need to have medication. Remember, too, that the dosage is usually reduced gradually. If you need pain medication while in the hospital, take it. You won't become a "drug addict" in a few short days, nor will your baby be adversely affected by it. If you don't need it, you have the right to refuse it. On the other hand, don't wait until you are so uncomfortable you can hardly see straight before asking for it. It won't work as effectively then.

Cesarean mothers should not compare their progress (nor be compared by others) with progress of a vaginally delivering mother, or in fact, with that of another cesarean mother. How quickly and easily one recuperates varies from woman to woman and even from one pregnancy to the next. The cesarean mother has special considerations and handicaps that must be taken into account.

One excellent innovation which some hospitals have introduced is the use of color-coded tags on the cribs of all babies delivered by cesarean. It is often impossible for nurses to remember which mothers had cesareans if there are many mothers on the maternity floor. These tags remind them that this mother and baby need extra time and attention. Tags on cribs automatically alert nurses to the fact that they will have to help the mother achieve a comfortable position for feeding (a pillow placed on the abdomen, and one or two under her back), and place the baby in the mother's arms before leaving the room. The nurse will also have to return to the mother's room within a few minutes to help her burp the baby and change sides for feedings. If the nurse does not return, the intercom or buzzer should be used—that's what they're there for.

Sometimes cesarean mothers are placed in rooms together and preferably in rooms closest to the nursery. Although it is not always possible, because of a "baby boom" or lack of beds, being with others who have shared a similar experience serves many useful purposes. For one thing, the cesarean mother won't be depressed when her roommate bounces out of bed minutes or hours after a vaginal delivery while she is still having trouble getting to and from the bathroom two, three, or four days after delivery. Cesarean mothers will be able to share their experiences and trade tips on how to deal with everything from the incision to the baby. Placing cesarean mothers in rooms closest to the nursery makes the walk less trying and tiring and will be especially appreciated those first few postpartum days. Many hospitals now have electric beds for all their patients. But when there are only a few available, it is thoughtful (and necessary) to save them for cesarean mothers. Being able to press a button to elevate her head or knees, or lower the bed so she can get out without having to call a nurse, is a small, but important consideration which also frees the nursing staff to do other things.

During the postpartum stay, the nursing staff or a special clinician may spend some time with cesarean mothers so they can talk about their experiences, ask questions, and relieve themselves of any psychological stress if they wish. If the mother was traumatized by the event, being able to talk about it will help her to sort out and work through any problems she may have. Negative experiences sometimes assume proportions far in excess of reality. If cesarean mothers are not afforded the benefits of someone to talk with, their impressions of the experience may become increasingly more bitter and horrifying.

Support groups, composed primarily of cesarean parents, are growing in number. Through these organizations, postpartum cesarean women are sometimes visited in the hospital. Although the woman who comes to visit will not be able to give medical advice (she does not need to—many doctors and nurses are on hand to fill this need), she will be able to listen and to talk with the mother about her own experiences and may help the new mother to cope with the myriad problems. It is important to erase the negative tapes playing in the minds of cesarean mothers, particularly those whose birth experiences have been anything but ideal. Emoting about the experience, in the company of someone who is empathetic and skilled at peer counseling, will benefit the new cesarean parent. What is needed and what is gained is an understanding of the emotional and physical aspects of the event from someone who has undergone a similar experience. If the cesarean mother feels isolated, frustrated, or has questions, this informal chat may be just the thing needed to overcome these feelings.

During the first few days after delivery, the new mother's body will change dramatically. After months of feeling like an overweight hippopotamus, the reduction in waist size is welcome. Like any new mother, cesarean women must wear those giant sanitary pads (euphemistically called "mouse mattresses"). Unless the hospital provides the kind of pads which have adhesive backing, a sanitary belt must be worn. Occasionally, the clasps on the belt bite into the skin. Using safety pins, rather than a belt, may be more comfortable. If you prefer tampons, ask your doctor how soon you can start using them. The lochia (vaginal discharge and bleeding), which continues for two to six weeks after delivery, is a good external indicator should internal problems arise. At any time during the postpartum period if the amount of flow increases, or if there are clots or an unusually foul smell, you should tell your doctor. (If you are at home, an increased flow usually means you are doing too much. Go to bed at once, prop your feet up, and let the dust and disorder accumulate.) Like women who deliver vaginally, it will be necessary for the cesarean mother to cleanse the perineal area each time she urinates for as long as the bleeding and discharge continue. This cleansing will reduce the chance of infection. Always wipe from front to back. (The anal and vaginal openings are very close together, so wiping from back to front may cause infection.)

In the hospital, cotton gowns are preferable to synthetic ones. Nylon and rayon cling and become easily twisted. Cotton gowns are also cooler. Hospitals are known to be over-heated, and the body of the new mother, which is going through a readjustment, may cause her to perspire profusely or have hot flashes. Finding pretty cotton gowns that open in the front—an important consideration for mothers who nurse their babies—is often difficult. If you can't find anything suitable in the sleepwear department, try substituting granny dresses, India print tunics, or at-home wear instead.

While you are in the hospital, try to get as much rest as pos-sible. Hospital routine, which includes frequent checks on vital signs, visits from the doctor, messengers bringing flowers and mail, bed baths or showers, room cleaning, changing the linen, and the bringing of medication, may inhibit, rather than promote rest. With all the necessary routines of the hospital, many women find that each time they doze off, someone else comes into the room. Closing the door and keeping a "No Visitors" or "Do Not Disturb" sign helps . . . sometimes. With a sign on the door, most people will at least knock. The mother may begin to feel that she will never get enough rest. She will, but it will take some time. Later on at home, she and baby can settle into their own beds, take the phone off the hook, enforce a "No Visitors" rule, and delegate the house-work to the father, grandmother, or friend.

Coughing, laughing, and sneezing may rekindle your fears about rupturing the incision. Because of surgery, medications, and confinement to bed (for at least twelve hours), you may find the desire to cough greater at this time. In an effort to guard the incision, you may try to suppress it. Don't. Instead, splint the incision with your hands and/or a pillow, then take a deep breath in, let it out, take another deep breath, and cough! Holding the cough back only makes matters worse. Coughing also promotes functioning of the lungs at full capacity again.

Some hospitals provide binders for cesarean mothers. A binder is a wide elastic belt that fits around the abdomen and is used for support. It may lessen the discomfort initially, but it has disadvantages. Two problems which may result are that the binder becomes a crutch and gives a false sense of security. It will also allow your abdominal muscles to relax rather than to tone and strengthen themselves. Weakened muscles will cause more discomfort in the long run and require a longer period for you to shape up and regain your figure. If it's absolutely necessary, use a binder, but do so judiciously. To promote better circulation, some doctors order support stockings or socks.

A minor annoyance following cesarean childbirth is itching of the incision. In fact, some women report that just thinking about the birth or hearing the word "cesarean" causes the scar to itch even months later. If itching is a problem, it may be helpful to scratch *another* part of your body. It just isn't polite to scratch the incision in some instances—especially if the incision is the lower segment type. Once the scar heals, baby oil may also relieve the itchiness. You can still wear a two-piece bathing suit or bikini, but you should block the sun's rays from the incision.

How well the scar heals depends primarily upon the mother's skin type. Standing straight and tall from the first time out of bed helps the skin incision to heal more neatly, too. Some skin types produce a raised, shiny, red scar, called a keloid formation, no matter how much care is taken. More often, the incision will fade almost totally, so that after a year or so, it is almost indiscernible. One advantage to the lower segment "bikini cut" is that after the pubic hair grows in, it becomes almost totally covered by the hair. One woman, who had planned an at-home delivery but who had to have a cesarean because the baby was breech and very large, said, "I never felt at all unattractive, even when the scar was fresh. It was like a merit badge. That's the way my beautiful baby decided to come into the world, so it didn't bother me at all, ever." Hers is a very positive attitude. There are other women who feel mutilated by the scar. Classical incisions are more likely to cause this type of resentment. The new mother may feel that she has become less attractive, and perhaps less sexually appealing to her mate. She may also worry that she will be unable to wear a bikini again. Nonsense. To be sure, the scar may cause some hesitation the first summer season, but it should not keep a woman out of a bikini if she has the figure for one anyway. Most people don't notice the scar at all, although the mother may think that it glares.

There will also be "The Day The Milk Came In," usually about the third postpartum day. Women with breasts the size of mosquito bites will look like voluptuous models. One's breast size is unrelated to one's ability to provide adequate milk to one's baby. What is important, is that your milk is nature's way of providing the perfect food for your baby. A hot water bottle or heating pad, a hot shower or wearing a bra for support, and patience will help to relieve any temporary discomfort caused by engorgement of the breasts. Nursing the baby will bring the greatest relief.

About the third day after delivery, the Blues may occur. The new mother may find herself in tears for no obvious reason—or for a trivial one. Perhaps the baby starts to cry just when the mother has just settled down for a nap. Being hungry may trigger the tears. The mother may be starving for "real" food. And there it is again: a tray full of gelatin, tea, and broth. The mother may hold back the tears (if she can) until the nurse leaves the room, and then the floodgates open. If the mother is feeling physically uncomfortable, the amount of depression may be magnified.

No matter what triggers the depression, the result is the same: the mother feels sad and miserable, or helpless and guilty. She *should* be happy (or so she tells herself) because everything is going well. The baby is healthy, beautiful, and hers at last. In a few days, she'll be going home. Normally, the mother is very independent. Now she must rely very heavily upon others to do things for her. So she cries. And woe to the father who comes to the hospital late on this day! His tardiness, however unintentional, is bound to make the mother feel even more sad and lonely. An understanding, loving father will accept the Blues with equanimity, and do everything he can to comfort his wife.

Although postpartum depression is usually no better or worse than for vaginally delivering mothers, there is one instance where the amount of postpartum depression may be greater for the cesarean mother. The mother who anticipated a shared vaginal delivery may be devastated by the unexpected turn of events. She had high expectations and had read or heard glowing accounts of the wonders and beauties of birth. She may have gone to prepared childbirth classes and diligently practiced the breathing exercises. She feels cheated and unhappy. The mother who has had a surprise cesarean may feel that her feminity has been undermined. She may think she has failed herself, her husband, her baby, perhaps even her instructor. She may resent her body for having let her down, her baby for complicating matters, the hospital staff for not supporting her sufficiently, or for giving her too much or too little medication. She's "failed" the test.

After a cesarean delivery, being unable to move effortlessly and being tired may also cause negative feelings. which may be compounded by seeing roommates who delivered vaginally at midnight have a complete breakfast and walk down to the nursery at 7 a.m. The cesarean mother may not have any of these feelings, or if she does, she may not articulate them or even acknowledge them. She needs extra support and encouragement from her mate and the hospital staff—but she may seem uncommunicative, or difficult to deal with.

Whatever the reason, postpartum depression can be very real and very traumatic. It may not surface until weeks later. It may be worse for the woman who delivers in the winter, when inclement weather "traps" her in the house for days at a time. Postpartum depression may not happen at all.

The physical stress of surgery, the demands of the newborn, the needs of the father and older children, the hormonal changes of going from pregnancy to nonpregnancy, singly or in combination, may create problems that range from "mild blues" to "severe anxiety or depression." Fatigue, trying to accomplish too much too soon, may increase the problem. The cesarean mother should give her body a chance to heal and remember that recovery physically and emotionally will come. It may take a few days or even weeks for full physical recovery and a return to emotional balance but it will happen. Women who are well-adjusted and delighted to be mothers can expect at least one or two "rocky" days when nothing seems to go right. The father's support, his participation in the mother's and baby's care, and a nursing staff that appreciates the special status of the cesarean mother will enable her to see things in a more positive perspective.

Rooming-in is possible for cesarean mothers—despite rumors to the contrary. The plan should be modified to partial rooming-in for the first few days so that the baby is with the mother only for short periods, rather than all day and all night. No matter how good the mother feels, she will tire quickly. She should not feel guilty if she wants to send the baby back to the nursery to that she can relax and nap. She will be a better mother if she is rested and comfortable. The quality of time spent with the baby is far superior to the quantity.

Three things that will speed recovery and allow cesarean mothers to take an active part in the care and feeding of their newborns are a supportive hospital staff, flexible policy, and Family-Centered Maternity Care. FCMC is, in essence, the

philosophy of regarding the mother, father, and baby as a unit.
To this end, fathers are encouraged to spend as much time as
they like at the hospital and to take an active role in caring for
the mother and baby. Even if this baby is the couple's second,
third, or fourth, the parents will want to familiarize themselves
with her unique personality, her unique rhythms, preferences,
and eccentricities before going home where there may be other
children who need tending and less time to spend with each
child individually. The father and mother who see their baby
born, who hold her within minutes of birth, who share the
joys and responsibilities of parenting are apt to be better
parents, able to relate to their baby in a very special way.

Separation of the family at the time of birth and during
the hospital stay is a fairly recent innovation. Until early in
this century, women gave birth at home. Slowly hospitals
gained favor, and "germs" became the byword and testament
of the medical profession. Mothers—and *especially* fathers—
became harbingers of contamination. Babies were placed in
sterile nurseries (which Ashley Montague says are so named
because nursing—that is, breastfeeding—is the only thing which
doesn't take place there) and brought to their mothers every
four hours for feeding: no more, no less. The babies' fussiness
and colic were blamed on mothers, rather than on the well-
intentioned but inhumane hospital routine. Visiting hours for
fathers were limited to an hour or two per day.

It is appalling to think that practices introduced in the 20's
should still be in effect in the 70's. In an effort to be "modern," some hospitals have missed the point of what is best for
the mother, father, and baby, who has come from a comfortable, warm, dark environment into the brightly lit nursery,
with its clear plastic cribs and prepackaged formulas. Blankets,
shirts, and diapers, no matter how well-washed and fabric-
softened, must scratch the newborn's tender flesh. Nurses,
however sweet, loving, and dedicated, cannot replace the
mother's arms and the familiar sound of her heartbeat and
voice.

Fortunately, many hospitals are now moving toward

Family-Centered Maternity Care. A hospital with Family-Centered Maternity Care may not describe its program with those exact words even though its program incorporates the elements of FCMC. Examples of FCMC policies are liberal visiting hours (often hospitals permit fathers to visit from 6 or 7 a.m. to 11 p.m.) or round-the-clock visitation to accommodate fathers with work schedules that don't permit them to come to the hospital during the day. In deference to "germs," the father is usually required to wear a hospital gown and sometimes a mask when the baby is in the mother's room. If the baby is not already in the room when he arrives, the father may go to the nursery for her. He can help make the mother comfortable for feedings, burp the baby, change diapers, or hold the child in his arms, study her features, count her fingers and toes, and do all the things fathers are supposed to and want to do.

Given the motivation and opportunity, the father is also a good coach who can remind the mother to do her abdominal tightening exercises, to get out of bed and stand straight, to lend an arm as she walks, brush her hair, help her get into the shower, stand by in case she becomes dizzy and needs help, rub her back, mop her brow, bring water and drinks, answer the phone, or run errands. These may seem like menial tasks, but the mother will very much appreciate them. These "little" things may tip the balance between a speedy recovery and one that is just mediocre. While many of these tasks can be accomplished by a nurse, the t.l.c. that only the father can give is what makes the difference.

Bath demonstrations, breastfeeding classes, and infant care programs are often open to fathers as well as mothers. These programs are usually offered several times a week (sometimes daily) but some hospitals do not have them. They are excellent ways of supporting and reassuring parents for taking care of baby at home.

Sometimes Family-Centered Maternity Care includes sibling visiting which allows older children to visit Mommy in the hospital. Little ones are eager to reassure themselves that

Mommy is all right, and they want to see their new little brother or sister. What used to be a "lump" in the mother's abdomen has become a little person who caused Mommy to go to the hospital. Is Mommy okay? What does the new baby look like? The "stranger" in the hospital becomes more of a reality and less of a threat when glimpsed first hand. Some parents fear that older children will cry and be sad when the time comes for them to leave Mommy and Baby in the hospital. It is probably better that older children see their mother and cry (if they are going to) than not to see her at all. More often than not, the older children will not cry when they leave. Usually it is the mothers who do! A child's sense of time is not as well-developed as an adult's. If the children are with Grandma or a friend, they'll probably be quite happy to leave Mommy to go home to watch a favorite television program or have an ice cream as a special treat. A long-range plus to sibling visiting is that most youngsters never visit hospitals unless they are admitted for illness or injury. Coming to the hospital at a time of happiness will make the hospital a less threatening place.

This new awareness of the special, different needs of cesarean families on the part of hospital staffs makes the difference between competent care and excellent, first-rate care. For the parents, this new understanding has special bonuses: they are delighted to discover that they are having better birth experiences and easier, more positive postpartum periods.

Going home is eagerly awaited. The new mother counts the days until she will be able to sleep in her own bed again, eat anything she wants to, and set up life with the new baby without the well-intentioned interruptions of hospital routines and schedules. If this is the parents' first baby, they may also feel the responsibilities of parenthood quite heavily. The new baby is so tiny, so helpless, and so dependent on the mother and father for nourishment and love. How can they possibly do the right things? Where do they go from here?

CHAPTER 13 THE "FOURTH" TRIMESTER

*W*HEN THE DAY for going home
arrives, the mother, for the first time in months, is able to don
a pair of jeans or slacks, or a dress of *approximately* the size
she used to wear before pregnancy enveloped her. (The word
"approximately" is intentional. It comes as a very discouraging
blow to some mothers to learn that they still have to wear
something looser than normal in order to allow for the increase in breast size and the still flabby belly.) The baby
is dressed in a brand-new outfit, especially selected for going
home. The father arrives at the hospital early to help get the
family organized and to sign the appropriate papers. If there is
a delay (either because the bill has not been computed, or because there is no one available to escort the mother and baby
to the car), the parents become jittery.

At last all is ready. The mother and father are safely seat-
belted, and the baby is placed in a car bed or seat designed for
safety. It is never too early to ensure the baby's well-being in
the car. Minor accidents can have disastrous consequences for
the baby held in the mother's lap.

Even if the ride home is short, the mother may be exhausted by the time they arrive. The excitement of going
home, dressing herself and the baby, and riding in the car may
wear her out. At home, older children or a proud grandmother
may be waiting. The mother finds that she is overjoyed to
greet her family and that the most comfortable spot for her

152

is in her own bed. Everything around her is familiar and reassuring. She and the baby settle down while the father and grandmother make lunch, play with older children, and cuddle the new baby. There is something very special and magical about a new baby. Every friend and relative within miles wants to get a close look as soon as possible. Their visits are often both welcome and taxing. At last the phone stops ringing, and the family settles down into a nice, happy routine—or so it is assumed.

If the baby is a first child, most parents envision this time of adjusting from couple to family in much the same way as family life is pictured on television commercials and magazine advertisements. The mother, father, and baby are always smiling. The baby is immaculately dressed, and the mother, beautifully coiffed and wearing a white designer gown, sits in a bentwood rocking chair. All is lovely, peaceful, and elegant. This is pure fantasy.

Then reality strikes. If your baby's gown was ever immaculate, you will learn that it does not remain so for long. Real babies have been known to spit up all over the designer creation, and even the most highly touted diapers, either from the diaper service or disposable, sometimes leak. The new parents may smile joyfully but not quite as often as those ads would have us believe. Dream babies, immaculate houses, elegant hairstyles and gowns, and reassuring, rhythmic schedules exist only in fantasies and dreams—and advertisements.

The "fourth" trimester is the first three months of the baby's life. Pregnancy is normally divided into three periods, called trimesters. These trimesters culminate in the birth of the baby, the end of pregnancy; but birth is not an end, it is a beginning. The "fourth" trimester is as crucial to the baby's development and well-being as the time she spends growing within the mother's uterus. It is also a time of change—often bordering on confusion and chaos—for the parents, who must adjust to their new roles, and the logistics of caring for the baby's needs. New parents, however much they love their baby, may be overwhelmed at times. The cesarean mother, whose energy reserves have been depleted, may discover that the fourth trimester is very demanding. It comes as a shock to parents to discover that their much-adored, beautiful infant has the lungs of Godzilla, the mouth of a hungry lumberjack, and the ability to go through more diapers in two days than they ordered for a whole week.

The first few months are the hardest for the parents. Both may be handicapped by lack of sleep, lack of time to be alone, and additional energy drains. Every action centers on the baby. It may seem that there are simply not enough hours in the day to care for the baby and fulfill the parents' needs as people. The mother, with her numerous roles of wife, lover, career person, and/or parent to other children, bears the brunt of the difficulties the first few months.

It is imperative that the cesarean mother have help at home for the first week or two. After the first two to six weeks, depending entirely upon the individual woman, the differences between the cesarean mother and the mother who has delivered vaginally are not so great. It's important to remember that the cesarean mother is mending her body from both childbirth and surgery. Regular household chores should be taken over by other family members. Fathers often plan to take time off when the baby is born so they can be at home that first week or two. Some fathers are able to obtain leaves of absence to fulfill the essential parenting role. Grandmothers, aunts, sisters. and friends usually volunteer to lend assistance. Ideally, the helper should be someone who is acceptable to both mother and father and whose help is welcomed. Some relatives, however well-intentioned, may create more problems than they solve. It's a sticky situation for the new parent who wishes to say no, but who does not want to hurt a relative's feelings. If there is no graceful way to refuse an eager but unwelcome grandparent or relative, the new parents may ask the person to come for a specific period. Knowing the person will leave on a certain day is comforting.

In the meantime, s/he will probably be as helpful as s/he can. More often than not, Grandmother's help is very much appreciated and the new family realize they could not have managed without her.

Above all, when friends ask, "What can I do?" ask them to prepare a meal that just needs to be heated and served. Friends would not offer if they didn't want to help. Making dinner for the new family will allow friends to feel helpful and will save your already overburdened energies.

If possible, prepare and freeze foods while you are pregnant for use after the baby is born. Leftovers make good "TV" dinners with dribs of this and that. If you can afford it, you may wish to send out for food. Even a pizza or sub makes a well-rounded meal when a salad is included. When you're feeling up to it, a restaurant dinner will make a welcome change of pace. *All* parents should be encouraged to go out to a favorite restaurant sometime before the baby is three or four weeks old. It will do wonders for the mother's morale. The father should be encouraged to help with meal preparations. He may claim he's a dunce in the kitchen, but both parents will survive quite nicely on prepared dinners heated and served by the father. Even a plate of scrambled eggs and ham, topped off with a fresh vegetable, and prepared by the father is welcome when the mother is feeling tired and hungry. For the first few weeks, use paper plates and plastic utensils. Their use is not ecologically sound, economical, or elegant, but it is helpful.

Bathing the baby can be done by the father and will provide him with a special sense of closeness to the baby. Fathers of breastfed babies welcome this opportunity to do something essential and comforting (which the mother could do), but which he enjoys doing. He may take special pleasure and pride in performing this task for the baby.

The new cesarean mother should not feel guilty if she wants to become a hermit for a few weeks. The telephone can be taken off the hook, and a "No Visitors, Please" sign posted on the door. One father placed such a sign on his door along with a list of chores that needed doing. Anyone who wanted to visit also helped with household tasks. As a new mother, you will need all your energy to cope with caring for yourself and the baby. When visitors do call, you may find it advantageous to remain in your gown and robe to remind visitors (and yourself!) that you should not become overtired. Loving and loved family or friends who stay too long and who do not respond to gentle hints can be told, "I'm sorry, you'll have to leave now. The doctor said Sally needs a lot of rest. It's time for her to take a nap. Won't you please come back in a few weeks?" Frequent rest breaks are advised. A rocking chair is soothing for both you and baby—and is a good exercise which does not require a lot of energy.

Restrictions on activities for the first six weeks after delivery depend primarily on the doctor's policies and any special medical circumstances that may arise. Some doctors discharge their patients from the hospital with no limitations. These mothers leave the hospital knowing they may drive a car, go skiing, or make love if they want to. The doctor who places no restrictions is banking on the mother's body and common sense to dictate her activities. The only drawback is that some women assume because their obstetricians told them they could do anything, that they will want to do everything. They won't. Top athletes may be able to go skiing within a week after delivery, but not many cesarean mothers will have the energy to climb two flights of stairs, much less ski down a mountain. The best thing to do is to take it easy and use common sense. Unfortunately, common sense is not always easy to find. Pressing yourself too hard, even if you have no restrictions, will make a longer recuperative period necessary. Do what you can—but don't overdo. And you should not feel guilty about being a little weak or becoming easily fatigued.

Just as there are doctors who place no limitations, the extreme conservative approach makes everything other than going to the bathroom and feeding the baby taboo. Common prohibitions may include any or all of the following:

No Driving. This limitation may be imposed for as little as one week after discharge from the hospital, up to the entire six-week period. The reasons are that the mother may still be weak and subject to dizzy spells. Driving also makes it easy for her to push herself to accomplish tasks for which she is not truly prepared, such as spending an hour at the supermarket or in a clothing store.

Limited Stair Climbing. If you live in a house where the only bathroom is on the second floor, to avoid climbing stairs you may wish to build a "nest" for yourself and the baby on the floor where the bathroom is located. Use a thermos or ice chest nearby to keep snacks for yourself and older children. It is much easier to keep a box of crackers stashed away in a bedroom than to have to go down to the kitchen each time your toddler or you want a snack. Carrot sticks, celery, cheese, raisins, and nuts are some other foods that are nutritious and can be prepared in advance and brought upstairs.

Not Carrying Heavy Objects. Heavy objects include laundry, groceries, and toddlers. Arrangements can be made for the father or a relative to do the marketing and laundry. What to do with a toddler who is unable to climb in and out of bed or up and down from a highchair unassisted is a definite problem. During pregnancy some parents prepare youngsters for the new baby's arrival by moving them from their cribs to a regular low bed. Some mothers train their children to step onto a chair before getting into and out of the crib with the sides lowered. The reason for the limitation on lifting heavy objects is that some doctors want their postpartum cesarean mothers to avoid exertion, but most doctors, being male, do not know what a real problem it creates for the mother who also has a toddler to contend with.

The incision should be completely healed within a few weeks after delivery. During those weeks the father or a helper will probably be around who can do most of the lifting. Rearranging the furniture is out, but hugging, kissing, and even lifting a toddler is not dangerous.

No Spicy Foods. This restriction is placed primarily on

mothers who must stay in bed most of the time because of other problems probably unrelated to the delivery. The purpose here is to reduce the possibilities of discomfort from gas. This limitation is also sometimes placed on nursing mothers. While limiting one's food is fine for upset stomachs, breastfeeding does not necessarily mean that the nursing mother will have to deprive herself of spices, garlic, onions, or chocolate. Think of the millions of women in Africa, Asia, and South America who eat such food as hot curries or chiles almost exclusively. Their babies do not seem to suffer. Experiment. If you and baby do not have problems with foods, then it is permissible to eat them.

No Tub Baths. Showers are usually permitted within a few days after delivery. Most houses and apartments have showers. For those places where showers are not available, one compromise is to fill the tub partially with water, and then get in and wash quickly. The mother may wish to sit on a safe, low stool or even an overturned plastic pan. The important thing is to avoid contamination of the vagina by the anal area while lochia (vaginal discharge) is still being produced.

The new cesarean mother should take a bath only when someone is in the house who can help out if she needs it. Dizziness, faintness, and hot flashes may continue for some weeks after the baby's birth. Especially at first, the mother may be stiff and welcome a helping hand into and out of the tub or shower. Any new mother may find it difficult to set aside time for grooming, and the cesarean mother, who is less agile, may have difficulty bending over the sink or may become dizzy standing in the shower long enough to shampoo her hair.

Once the lochia has ceased, the baby may be taken into the bath with the mother. Fathers can take the baby into the bath after the umbilical cord has healed and dropped off, which usually occurs within the first week or two of the baby's life.

No Sex for Six Weeks. The intention is to reduce the

possibilities of infection, although some authorities believe
the taboo comes more from Judeo-Christian tradition than
from established medical fact. Many things other than penetration of the vagina by the penis constitute lovemaking and
can be equally satisfying. If you cannot wait to have intercourse, two things should be kept in mind. (1) You are not
alone. There are many other couples who cannot wait for the
go-ahead from the doctor which will be given at the six-week
checkup. Also, a red flag will not go up during the examination to signal your transgression to the doctor—but most
women confess to this "sin," even if somewhat sheepishly.
(2) Even though you may not have had a period, you may still
ovulate. Birth control should be used. If you are breastfeeding,
a diaphragm or condom are best. Breastfeeding mothers
cannot take the Pill when nursing. The diaphragm, if used,
must be well lubricated with spermicidal jelly, because it may
not fit properly. Be prepared! (See section on "Sex and the
Cesarean Couple" later in this chapter.)

Both mothers and babies are scheduled for checkups soon
after delivery. Usually few complications occur between the
hospital discharge and the postpartum visit. If there are
any problems or questions, call the obstetrician.

Although six weeks is a reasonable time for the first check-
up, there is a growing and positive trend for babies to have
their first visit with the pediatrician within two to four
weeks after birth. Although new parents should feel free to
call the pediatrician at any time, many parents have not yet
established a rapport with the baby's doctor and feel hesitant
about telephoning for fear of appearing "foolish" and "nervous" for being concerned about a rash, a change in bowel
movements, or recurrent spitting up. There is a certain reassurance that comes with visiting the pediatrician. Even if
the couple are "old pros" at parenting, all new parents worry
and fret over every diaper rash, flaky scalp, and change in
the baby's eating and sleeping habits. Seeing the pediatrician at two or three weeks will set many of the parents'

fears to rest before they become blown out of proportion and will stem any potentially serious problems before they become full-fledged.

Parents and babies who deliver at hospitals where policies are restrictive and unsupportive, and where Family-Centered Maternity Care is unknown, will want to implement their own family-centered touching and bonding program when they get home. Going home may be the first time the father has been able to see his baby without having to stare through a plate glass window. It may be the first time he has been able to hold her. The new mother, who has been able to have her baby only for short periods at four-hour intervals, may have little inkling of her baby's personality, feeding patterns, and sleeping habits. Breastfeeding may have been difficult to manage under such circumstances, especially in hospitals where babies are fed supplements regardless of the parents' wishes. Instead of going home with confidence and knowing what the baby is like, these parents are suddenly thrust into parenthood without preparation. The baby may be fretful at home, even though she never seemed to cry while in the hospital. If medical problems have been ruled out as the cause of the baby's problem, the child may need extra love and touching.

By all means, bring the baby into bed with you. Does this mean that *all* babies who are held and touched will automatically stop crying and go to sleep? No. A fretful baby who will not sleep in a way the parents think is "proper" is the source of a great deal of worry to them. Crying may simply be the baby's way of making her presence known. Cesarean babies, who more often than not have been separated from their mothers for varying time periods, need *extra* body contact the first few days and weeks. The parents who take a baby home from the hospital where little contact has been allowed will want to give their babies additional touching, stroking, nuzzling, kissing, and cuddling. Although it is sometimes considered unfashionable by modern standards, once home from the hospital, the best place for the mother and baby the first week at home is in bed *together*. The more frequently the baby is offered the warmth and closeness of the mother's body (and to a lesser degree, the father's body, too), the more secure the baby will feel.

A happy, secure, contented baby will not cry often. Despite our hang-ups, the fact is that holding and cuddling a baby will *not* spoil her. The baby needs attention. Crying is the only way she has to get it. It may take a few weeks for the parents to determine what the baby is "saying." Sometimes it means "feed me," other times the cry means, "I'm wet and want to be changed" (although it does seem odd that a baby who has spent nine months in a wet world would mind being damp provided she is *warm*), and sometimes it just means, "I need attention. Please love me." A baby carrier, fashioned of any soft, comfortable material, or purchased (a "Snugli" is one excellent baby carrier), will make the baby feel secure and will leave the mother's hands free to do whatever she wants.

No matter what the parents do, there will be times when the baby's crying turns the parents' rose-colored glasses purple with rage. Acceptance of the fact that the infant is almost sure to cause chaos at home for a few months will help the parents deal with the situation more realistically. There will be times when the parents are able to enjoy a nice, quiet evening together while the baby slumbers peacefully. At first, however, these times of tranquility may be few and far between. They are outnumbered by the daily hassles of dirty diapers, a hungry baby, and the usual, never-ending household chores. Maintaining a semblance of dignity and personhood is often difficult for new parents to attain.

There are benefits and joys to parenting. Most of the burden rests on the mother, and she is the one most apt to receive the benefits, but unfortunately they are not as numerous or apparent initially as the negative aspects. The circles under your eyes will disappear. You will be able to get a long, uninterrupted night's sleep . . . sometime—and, with luck, soon. There

will be a time when you can pick up and take off for an out-
ing without enough equipment and strategy-planning for an
African safari. And you will be able to make love spontaneously without being interrupted by the baby's cries . . . sometime. At first, however, the baby takes precedence. To add to
these frustrations, if you think that a really good mother or
father *never* temporarily resents the baby's intrusion, your
frustration may be compounded by guilt. Even the world's
best mothers and fathers sometimes experience any or all of
the feelings of frustration, anger, or resentment that a new
baby may create.

To help you smooth over the "fourth" trimester, there are
a number of good books available. The best rule of thumb
when reading books on child care is to use them as a guide.
The best points of each must be assimilated into your family's
life-style and the personality of your baby.

Each baby and each parent are different. Change, chaos,
disorder, and confusion are all normal conditions those first
few months. Learn to flow with the river—don't try to push
it. It's hard to believe that a tiny infant can create such havoc
with an otherwise stable household. Let the dust accumulate
and take the time to enjoy your baby. Cultivate the services
of a good, reliable sitter, and treat yourself to an afternoon
off. When you come back, you'll probably feel rejuvenated.

The father who shares in the responsibilities of caring for
the children and house will gain a special closeness to his
children. Both father and baby have the need and right to be
with each other. A warm, loving relationship will flourish.
Some fathers offer to take over all the responsibilities for an
evening or afternoon, thus allowing the mother time to herself. She needs this time and will appreciate the father's caring.
It may help to promote a new awareness of their relationship
with each other. Today's fathers are spending more time with
infant care. They are aware of the fact that tenderness does
not mean a lack of manliness, but rather is a reflection of
their "humanness." (And mothers, if dad does take over the

Baby Equipment and Clothing

That old Yankee saying, "Use it up, wear it out, make it do, or do without" seems all but lost in our disposable, throw-away, plastic society. Everything from automobiles to diapers is designed with obsolescence in mind.

It isn't necessary to spend hundreds (sometimes thousands) of dollars on the newest, biggest, best, shiniest baby equipment and clothing. You can outfit your baby and provide for all her furniture needs without spending a fortune.

Baby equipment and furniture can be swapped or borrowed. Classified ads in local newspapers and bargain weeklies are good sources. Yard, barn, and garage sales are excellent places to purchase used baby items for a mere fraction of their original cost.

Baby clothes can also be found in yard sales, flea markets, and thrift shops. Check the clothing over carefully because sometimes it is stained and ripped. If you don't mind, your baby won't. A complete, attractive layette can usually be purchased. When cleaned it will look as though it came from the town's most expensive store.

The two most important items your baby will need are a firm mattress and a safe car carrier. The car seat should be sturdy and face toward the back of the car when installed. A worn, too-soft mattress is bad for the infant's soft, rapidly growing bones. A piece of foam 2 or 3 inches thick makes an excellent, inexpensive mattress, can be cut to any size or shape, and is ideal if you've just bought a delightful but eccentrically shaped antique crib or cradle.

Strollers, musical swings, cribs, cradles, mobiles, back carriers, and all other items are usually readily available—although some items are more in demand than others (a used Snugli is hard to find), so you may have to shop around a bit. You'll be saving money and recycling at the same time!

cooking, cleaning, baby care, or laundry, let him do it *his* way. It may be different from your way but that doesn't matter.)

Be sure to take time out for yourself as a "person" and yourselves as a "couple." Do things you enjoy doing together. If someone offers to take the baby for a few hours or help out with the house, don't refuse this offer. Don't overlook your responsibilities to yourselves. Leave the baby with Grandma or a friend and do something special, just the two of you. If you don't have a close friend or relative to take the baby for a few hours, it may be possible to arrange a "swap" with a friend. You spend a certain number of hours with her baby in exchange for a few of her hours with yours.

At one time or another, most parents say, "I could just throw the kid out the window, I'm so mad." But if that is the only way they feel, or if they say they want to do away with the child and really mean it, professional help is imperative. If the aggravations of parenthood are overwhelming or persistent, professional counseling is advised.

Many communities now offer groups for the education and support of new parents. They may be postpartum groups that have developed as an outgrowth of a prepared childbirth program, or they may have formed as the result of parental interest. Some of these groups have regular meetings as well as supplemental hot lines or listening ear services. When a parent feels ready to "blow up," a phone number is dialed and negative feelings, questions or concerns may be vented to the person at the other end of the line—instead of at the baby. If there is no such program in your area, a friend may be able to help.

For first-time parents, this chapter may seem unnecessarily gloomy. Veteran parents will be aware of the realities and responsibilities of caring for a newborn. Parenthood is an awesome responsibility. "Real" babies are wonderful and precious. They also wet, cry, get hungry, sleep (but not always at the most convenient hours), and fret. There is pleasure and joy which comes from holding the baby in your arms. There is pride and happiness when the baby smiles at you for the first time. There is something very special and fulfilling about seeing part of you reflected in your baby's features and habits. Once you've made it through the first three or four months, you will probably forget—or at least gloss over—the trials and tribulations of this fourth trimester.

SEX AND THE CESAREAN COUPLE

As a new mother, you may find that your interest in sex is at an all-time low. Childbirth via surgery, the demands of the newborn, the lack of a full night's sleep without interruption for at least one feeding, and caring for the house and older children as well as the new baby may be so draining that you have neither the time nor the inclination to make love, at least for a while. The baby's father may not be the type to pressure you about sex, but you may pressure yourself into wanting to please your partner, even though you're not feeling up to it. After all, he has not had a baby, so his level of desire is not affected.

Some couples do make love either with or without the doctor's permission before the six weeks are up. The woman's vagina may not lubricate as well as it did before she had the baby. Lack of lubrication is a normal course of events brought about by the hormonal changes of giving birth, but it may cause discomfort or pain. Vaseline, K-Y Jelly, or any other brand of lubricant rubbed on the penis or vagina, or both, before intercourse will overcome the lack of lubrication and make penetration easier.

During pregnancy it is a good idea to explore how you will deal with contraception afterward. Birth control is necessary if you wish to space your pregnancies and are not ready for permanent sterilization. Finding a suitable temporary method is difficult. Prior to the six-week checkup, the mother who wants to use an IUD will not have had one inserted. A dia-

phragm that fit properly before pregnancy may not offer the
same amount of protection now, for the opening in the
cervix can stretch somewhat during pregnancy even in cesarean mothers. If you do use your old diaphragm, be sure
to apply lots of spermicidal jelly. Condoms are acceptable
methods of birth control, although some people find them
distasteful and/or do not like them because they may reduce
sensation. Withdrawal before ejaculation is not satisfactory,
because the risk is that sperm may be present in pre-ejacula-
tory fluid. Foams and spermicidal jelly used singly are
anything but fail-safe. Birth control pills, of course, cannot
be taken by nursing mothers because the hormones they contain will be transmitted to the baby. Plan ahead!

The mother's scar can be a source of concern. Won't it be
ruptured making love? Does it make the woman less appealing
to her mate? The classical cesarean skin incision from belly
button to pubis is particularly blatant. The woman's pubic
hair has been shaved, and she may feel like a plucked chicken,
which further lowers her morale. As the pubic hair grows
back, it itches or prickles, a sensation which may be irritating
as she rubs her body against her mate's. The newly delivered
cesarean mother feels particularly vulnerable at this time,
when her incision is fresh and her pubic hair shorn. Rupture of
the scar is all but impossible, but its presence is a reminder
to both the mother and father that this is a time to be gentle
and considerate.

Women's concerns about the scar are sometimes valid. A
very few are initially repulsed by it. Most men are understanding and accept it with even greater ease than the mother
herself. The best thing for the couple to do is talk about their
feelings openly and honestly soon after the baby is born. The
"problem" may not be a problem at all, except in the mother's
mind. She meeds reassurance that she is no less lovely and
appealing than before.

Making love can be relaxing and fulfilling—at a time when
the mother and father are able to share the closeness and

warmth that can only be expressed sexually—or it can be a time of resentment and frustration for both partners. If the mother feels pressured into making love before she is ready, if the baby starts to fuss right in the middle of things, the mother is apt to be so distracted that her mind wanders.

The baby's father needs to exhibit patience, understanding, and tact—but he may find these concerns for the mother's welfare difficult to express if he has been unable to fulfill his desire for weeks or even months. Few doctors, except in special cases, routinely prohibit sex during the last six weeks of pregnancy, but there are exceptions.

During pregnancy the mother may have felt more amorous than usual. After the baby is born her desire to make love may be lessened. This temporary decrease is partially due to physical fatigue from the stress of surgery, childbirth, and the extra demands the new baby places on her time and energy. It is normal, it is natural, but it can be disturbing to both parents. The father may secretly resent the baby for intruding and requiring so much attention. The mother may have these feelings, too.

Finding the time to make love may require more planning and cooperation than it did before. And the parents may wish to express their love in other forms of pleasuring rather than intercourse. Getting back to "normal" may take time, but it can be achieved. Understanding on the part of both parents will make this transition easier.

POSTPARTUM EXERCISES

The cesarean mother is apt to believe that her stomach muscles have been severed and that she can never hope to have a flat stomach again. This myth is widespread, inaccurate, and convenient—why exercise when it won't help anyway?

Right after delivery, the new mother may feel like Twiggy. However, when she gets on the scales at home, or tries to put on a comfortable pair of slacks, she may realize that she isn't quite as thin as she thought she was. It takes at least a few weeks for her to lose every ounce of weight gained during pregnancy, and even if she does get back to prepregnancy size, there may still be some extra, very discouraging flab in the way.

You should discuss any diet planned for weight loss and an exercise program designed for reducing flab and extra inches with your doctor. Generally, once the mother has had her six-week check-up, it is safe to begin an exercise program. In the meantime, the mother can use a rocking chair to promote circulation and, after a week or so when she is less bothered by the incision, she can "walk" by pressing her feet against a pillow at the end of her bed while pulling her stomach in and letting it out at the same time. This exercise also promotes circulation and will help the muscles of the abdomen tone up. The abdominal tightening exercise will help, too.

After your obstetrician has given the go-ahead, almost any exercise program is acceptable. Some organizations offer classes in swimming, slimnastics, and postpartum exercises. Walking, bike riding, tennis, and jogging (with the doctor's all-clear signal) also promote muscle tone. Doing sit-ups, deep knee bends, and running-in-place will also help. Just be certain to check with your doctor and don't overdo any exercises.

CHAPTER 14 HUMAN BONDING: THE IMPORTANCE OF TOUCHING AND THE ADVANTAGES OF BREASTFEEDING

Caesarean-delivered babies suffer from a number of disadvantages from the moment they are delivered. . . .

It may be conjectured that the disadvantages, among other things, from which caesarean-delivered babies suffer, compared with vaginally delivered babies, are to a significant extent related to the failure of adequate cutaneous stimulation which they have undergone. . . .

The moment it is born, the cord is cut or clamped, the child is exhibited to its mother, and then it is taken away. . . .

The two people who need each other at this time, more than they will at any other in their lives, are separated from one another, prevented from continuing the development of a symbiotic relationship which is so crucially necessary for the further development of both of them.

During the whole of pregnancy the mother has been elaborately prepared, in every possible way, for the continuation of the symbiotic union between herself and her child, to minister to its dependent needs in the manner for which she alone is best prepared. It is not simply that the baby needs her, but that both need each other. The mother needs the baby quite as much as the baby needs its mother. The biological unity maintained by the mother and conceptus throughout pregnancy does not cease at birth but becomes—indeed, is naturally designed to become—even more intensified and interoperative than during utero-gestation. Giving birth to her child, the mother's interest and involvement in its welfare is deepened and reinforced. Her whole organism has been readied to minister to its needs, to caress it, to make loving sounds to it, to nurse it at the breast. . . .

During the birth process mother and infant have had a somewhat trying time. At birth each clearly requires the reassurance of the other's presence. The reassurance for the mother lies in the sight of her baby, its first cry, and in its closeness to her body. For the baby it consists in the contact with and warmth of the mother's body, the support in her cradled arms, the caressing it receives, and the suckling at her breast, the welcome to the "bosom of the family." These are words, but they refer to very real psycho-physiological conditions.[1]

Modern science is just now recognizing what so-called primitive cultures have known and practiced for centuries: that the newborn human infant needs to be stroked and touched as much as she needs to be nourished and kept warm. If she is to develop into a happy, secure, intelligent person, it is important to keep the parents (especially the mother) and baby together as much as possible from the moment of birth and to offer the opportunity for them to have early, frequent, close physical contact. These are not "niceties." They are essential.

"Human bonding" is the term used by professionals for the very complex processes that establish deep and lasting emotional ties between parents and their offspring. Many assume that parental love comes in an immediate, intense, blinding, automatic, almost magical flash. It doesn't. The first few days and weeks of the infant's life, extending for the next six to nine months, is a crucial period when the roots of love are planted. From these roots, the child will flourish or fail to thrive. Human bonding is a period of adjustment, a sort of ritual recognition, a "welcome to the world" ceremony with both immediate and long-range consequences. Early, frequent contact between the parents and baby will lay the foundation for the nurturing and care of the baby's physical and emotional needs. Bonding is a term which encompasses acceptance of the baby by the parents (and vice versa), the way the parents and baby relate to each other, and the *quality* of the care extended to the baby. The baby who is loved, stroked, admired, gazed at, talked to, held close, and cuddled is the child who will thrive and who will grow into a secure, well-adjusted adult human being.

Babies pick up "messages" from parents. These messages

may be verbal ("oohing" and "aahing," cooing, or singing a lullaby are positive messages; a harsh, loud voice is a negative one) or tactile (the infant can sense from the way she is handled whether the "message" or "vibe" is positive or negative). The baby who is born into a warm, demonstrative atmosphere with a significant person, usually the mother, lavishing affection on her, will have a firm foundation on which to build future human relationships. Many factors determine the quality of the initial contact between the mother and baby. This initial contact is of great importance. Yet for the cesarean family, outside influences may greatly hinder or impede the establishment of parental-infant bonding. For example, an emergency cesarean, performed after a long and difficult labor, will have depleted the mother's energy reserves. Her physical and emotional condition (for example, if she is in great pain, frightened, or confused by the events around her) will inhibit the maternal-infant bonding process. This reaction is understandable, and the mother is justified in being somewhat more egocentric than she would have been had the labor and delivery taken place easily. If the delivery has taken place with general anesthesia, it will be many hours before the mother and baby are united. Even if spinal or epidural anesthetic has been used, the mother whose baby is whisked away with only a fleeting glimpse (or none at all) will not be able to initiate the maternal-infant bonding and attachment processes immediately as is ideal. When parents and babies are separated for many hours or days, the bonding process is delayed. Hospitals with rigid four-hour feeding schedules, and limited Family-Centered Maternity Care (if it is provided at all) hinder the bonding and touching rituals.

It is usually easier to initiate the bonding and touching processes in a vaginal delivery. To illustrate, here is a description of an "ideal" vaginal delivery (and few vaginal deliveries are as easy and straightforward as the one presented here).

The "ideal" vaginal delivery takes place after a 12-hour labor in which the mother has had no medication. She has been comfortable and in control of the situation by using one of the breathing methods (such as

Bing, Lamaze, or Kitzinger) learned in prenatal classes. Her husband has been with her throughout labor as coach and supporter, and he comes with her to the delivery room. Within seconds of birth, the infant is held up for the parents to see before the umbilical cord is cut. The infant is placed on the mother's abdomen for this process. Then the child is cared for beside the parents. As soon as the nurse has tended to the baby, she is presented to the mother and father for touching and admiration. Within minutes the baby is put to the mother's breast.

The parents and their baby are the center of attention. All the doctors and nurses congratulate the parents and praise the infant for her beauty, her lusty cry, or her plumpness. The parents and baby are taken to the recovery room, and the next few hours are spent admiring the baby, stroking her, kissing her, rubbing her body gently, and holding her close. The mother then rests for a short time, and full rooming-in begins later that day or early the next morning. The father comes to the hospital frequently and helps to care for and caress the baby. The baby is fed on demand, when she is hungry, not according to some preordained schedule.

The mother and baby go home from the hospital within three or four days. The child is not relegated to a separate room, but kept in the parents' room. At night, the parents have no hesitation about bringing the baby into bed with them, knowing that parents have an "automatic alarm" system that prevents them from rolling over on the baby. When the baby awakens at night for feedings, the father changes the baby and the mother has only to turn on her side or prop herself up on pillows to feed the baby. No chilly trips to the kitchen, no waiting for a bottle to heat. Usually the baby falls asleep in the mother's arms, and she can simply lay the child down before she falls asleep again.

During the day, the baby is frequently carried about in a backpack or front carrier. The mother's hands are free, and she can walk, vacuum, read, or tend to her plants easily and comfortably. The baby, meanwhile, is reassured by the closeness of the mother's body, the sound of her familiar heartbeat and voice. On weekends, the family take hikes or bike trips with the baby safely strapped to a backpack. The father spends several hours a day with the baby, changing diapers, talking with her, playing with her, bathing her. On weekends, he encourages the mother to spend several hours at the library, digging in the garden, or visiting a museum while he takes over the baby's care.

How does this idealized illustration of a vaginal delivery and postpartum period compare to the average cesarean experience? Usually the parents are separated for the cesarean birth, and perhaps for many hours afterward. The baby is not shown

to the mother, but taken immediately from the delivery room
and down to the special care nursery where the child will remain for at least 12 to 24 hours. The mother, unable to move
easily and comfortably for two or three days, must depend
heavily on the nursing staff for her care as well as for her
baby's. Unless the mother has special time and attention,
breast-feeding will be difficult for her to initiate. She must
have help, either from the staff or the baby's father, in getting
positioned for feedings, changing sides, and burping and
diapering the baby. At home, she will be unable to carry the
baby about for at least a few weeks, because the incision,
and her fatigue, will make it almost impossible.

What can parents and hospital personnel do to improve the
situation for cesarean families? How can early, frequent
bonding and touching be established for these parents and
babies? Some suggestions for more positive approaches and
more supportive care, which have already been instituted in
a growing number of hospitals, are:

1. Ideally, unless there are medical contraindications, the
mother should be awake for the baby's birth. Being awake
will enable her to establish immediate contact with the infant.
Seeing one's baby is a right, not a privilege. The baby is not
"hospital property."

2. If the umbilical cord is long enough, the obstetrician
could hold the baby up high enough over the screen so the
mother can see her seconds-old baby all wet and covered with
vernix. Parents have envisioned this moment for many years,
and their desire to see it has been reinforced by books, films,
and articles. It is a precious sight and one to which cesarean
parents are entitled.

3. Cesarean parents should be permitted to witness the birth
together. This sharing will strengthen their sense of togetherness and will establish and promote parental-infant bonding.

4. The nurse or pediatrician should give the mother a quick
glimpse of the baby before the infant is placed in the baby-
warmer unit. It is important to resuscitate the baby, clean

mucus from it mouth, give additional oxygen, take her Apgar rating, and keep the child warm, so a quick view of the baby can take place as the child is en route to the baby-warmer unit.

5. The baby unit should be placed within eyesight of the mother. After months of waiting for this day, seeing the back of someone's head and hearing "Your baby is fine" will not do. Only the sight of her baby will reassure her.

6. As soon as the baby has been immediately cared for, she should be presented to the mother for eye and skin contact. Although the cesarean mother's hands are usually not free, she can touch the baby with her face. This kissing, nuzzling, touching, stroking, and smelling will release the mother's maternal responses and will reassure her.

7. The father, if he is present, can cuddle the baby close and talk with the mother for 5, 10, or 15 minutes before the baby is taken to the nursery. If the father is not present, a nurse or the pediatrician will have to act as the "significant other."

8. Most states require that silver nitrate or a similar solution be administered to the eyes of all newborns. Some medical professionals now believe that delaying the administration of eyedrops is advantageous in that it allows the mother and baby to see each other and the eye drops can be administered in the nursery just as easily as in the delivery room.

9. For parents who wish to have a Leboyer delivery, it is possible to achieve the spirit of this method with gentleness, warmth, soothing voices, and stroking, although dim lights and massage of the infant on the mother's abdomen are not possible.

10. Reuniting parents and babies in the recovery room as soon as possible—as soon as the baby has been examined and her temperature has stabilized at normal—will release many of the maternal responses and will reassure the parents. For

the infant, being held in the mother's arms will replicate the warmth and reassurance of the intrauterine environment and will promote closeness and security.

11. The condition of cesarean babies should be judged on an individual basis. Until recently, all cesarean babies were placed in the special care nursery for observation regardless of their birth weight, Apgar score, temperature, or overall condition. This tradition sprang from the high incidence of respiratory distress among cesarean-delivered babies. Now, thanks to prenatal tests to determine fetal maturity and well-being, and improved medical, surgical, and neonatal techniques and equipment, the cesarean baby has a greater-than-ever opportunity to be born healthy and full term.

Parents should consult with a pediatrician before delivery to determine what policies their hospitals and doctors have. Engaging the services of a sympathetic pediatrician in advance of delivery may enable you to have and to hold your healthy, unendangered baby soon after delivery—rather than hours or days later. While no one would advocate anything but the best care for an endangered infant, it is now possible to have a perfectly healthy cesarean baby who does not need the special care nursery.

12. Giving the mother an opportunity to begin breastfeeding soon after birth will give the baby the benefit of skin contact and colostrum.

13. During the family "reunion" in the recovery room, the staff will want to maintain a low profile, and to intrude only if the parents ask for assistance or advice.

14. Where central nurseries, separate from the maternity floor or recovery room, are used, the mother needs constant assurances from the staff and the baby's father that her child is alive and well. This reassurance is just as important for mothers who have been reunited with their infants in the recovery room as it is for those who cannot have and hold

their babies for many hours. An instantly developed picture of the child will reassure her further.

15. Once the mother has begun rooming-in (and later at home) she may wish to keep the room fairly dim for the baby who has lived for nine months in a warm, dark world. Rocking chairs, unfortunately not found in most American hospitals, are soothing and relaxing for mother and baby.

16. Fathers should be encouraged, through flexible, accommodating hospital policies, to take part in caring for and nurturing their infants. Support from the hospital staff with a "it's so nice you're here" attitude (as opposed to "fathers are always in the way") will promote the father's attachment to the child.

If the cesarean family is unable to establish immediate eye and skin contact, or cannot care for the child as they would like to in the hospital because of medical reasons or hospital practice, they should reassure themselves that they will be able to make up for lost time and nurture the child according to their own wishes once they are home. A parent who is highly motivated will overcome any obstacle.

And the baby who is loved and cherished, touched and kissed will thrive. It has been said that the price we human beings pay for our higher intellect is a loss of instinct. This seems to be particularly true with regard to current birthing practices and child care attitudes. But the tide is turning. Parents are beginning to trust themselves and their instincts more. Your baby knows what she wants and needs. And you know how to provide it. Some things have to be learned—such as how to fasten a diaper securely on a wiggling baby—but most things will come automatically. If our babies could talk, they might say, "See me, feel me, touch me, love me."— and that's just what many parents are doing. They're looking at their babies, talking with them, carrying them about in backpacks or front carriers, holding them close in their arms, bringing the baby into bed with them, breastfeeding them, and doing all the things babies need and want. As parents, we want

to give our babies the best possible start in life. A healthy
human being is not just one who cries at birth and who "pinks
up" rapidly, but one who as an adult is physically, neurologi-
cally, and emotionally sound. And the ways to achieve that
well-being begin at birth. Not everything can be measured in
quantitative scientific terms. In human terms, touching and
bonding will improve the quantity and quality of the life of
the human child.

It is through body contact with the mother that the child makes its
first contact with the world, through which he is enfolded in a new
dimension of experience, the experience of the world of the other.
It is this . . . that provides the essential source of comfort, security,
warmth, and increasing aptitude for the new experiences. . . .

What the child requires if it is to prosper . . . is to be handled and
carried, caressed and cuddled, and cooed to, even if it isn't breastfed.
It is handling, the carrying, the caressing and that cuddling that we
would here emphasize, for it would seem that even in the absence of a
great deal else, these are the reassuringly basic experiences that the
infant must enjoy if it is to survive in some semblance of health. Extreme
sensory deprivation in other respects, such as light and sound, can be
survived, as long as the sensory experiences of the skin are maintained.

To be tender, loving and caring, human beings must be tenderly loved
and cared for in their earliest years, from the moment they are born.
Held in the arms of their mothers, caressed, cuddled, and comforted,
the familiar human environment . . . is found. . . .[2]

WHY BREASTFEEDING MAY BE OF SPECIAL SIGNIFICANCE TO CESAREAN MOTHERS AND BABIES

Breastfeeding is not only *possible* after a cesarean delivery; in
my view, it is often preferable for cesarean mothers and
babies.

Rarely are cesarean mothers too weak or infants too ill to
be breastfed. The "problems" associated with breastfeeding
come primarily from societal attitudes that there is something
"dirty" or "old-fashioned" about it. Hospitals are not immune
to those pressures and may have restrictive policies that re-

strain rather than encourage and promote breastfeeding. The
new mother has many questions about feeding her baby. To
overcome any hesitation she may have, she needs information,
encouragement, and understanding. The mother who asks
her obstetrician, nurse, or pediatrician about breastfeeding
does not want to hear, "Well, you can if you want to. It's

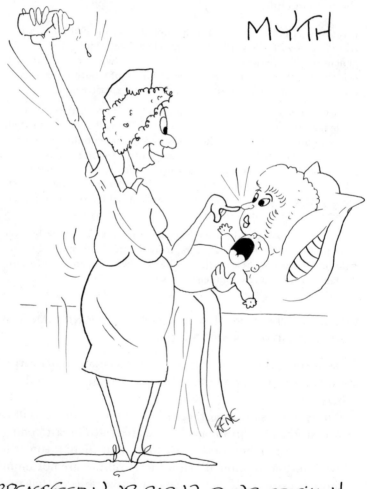

MYTH

BREASTFEED YOUR BABY? DON'T BE SILLY!
DON'T YOU KNOW SECTION WOMEN CAN'T?

really up to you." She knows that already. She wants information. She may need only a bit of encouragement to convince her that breastfeeding is proper, best for her baby, and natural. Doctors and nurses who feel comfortable discussing breastfeeding and respond with, "Of course you want to know about it. It's best for you and baby . . ." are to be commended. Unfortunately many health care professionals are just as confused and uptight as some parents. Often the most positive, informative assistance the new or expectant mother can obtain comes from groups such as La Leche League, an organization with chapters in many cities and towns throughout the country. Any parent interested in learning more about breastfeeding is encouraged to attend a meeting of a local chapter or write to La Leche League Headquarters at 9616 Minneapolis Avenue, Franklin Park, Illinois 60131. You don't have to become a member to attend local meetings. La Leche League is the best and often the only place where parents can turn to find out about breastfeeding.

In the United States, an estimated 10 to 25 percent of the mothers breastfeed their babies. This low statistic is both shocking and disquieting. Why so few? Who or what is to be blamed? And what are the special advantages of breastfeeding as they apply to the cesarean mother and baby?

The cesarean baby, who has not had the beneficial stimulation of labor, who has not passed through the birth canal, and who has probably been separated from the mother immediately after birth, has special handicaps. To make up for these handicaps, cesarean babies may need the mother's milk even more than vaginally delivered babies—although breastfeeding is certainly the best way to nourish any infant.

Breastfeeding, in addition to its nutritional benefits, is a natural intimate relationship between mother and baby. If the mother feels uncomfortable with her body or its functions, she may find breastfeeding difficult—if not impossible. One slogan of our era should be, "Let's get our breasts out of the pages of girlie magazines and into our babies' mouths where they belong!" It is because of this emphasis on breasts as sex symbols and objects of fantasy (rather than sources of nourishment and comfort to our children) that many now regard breastfeeding as "smutty." Mothers who breastfeed their babies may find it absurd—if not vulgar—to watch a mother shove a plastic bottle into a baby's mouth. Yet many others are conditioned to think that it is pornographic to use breasts for their natural function. How sad.

One distinct advantage to breastfeeding is that it sets up a built-in system of immunizing the baby against many diseases. This immunization begins with the first few drops of colostrum the baby takes the first time she nurses.

A disadvantage of not breastfeeding is that "menstrual bleeding tends to be heavier and longer-lasting when the mother does not breastfeed, and, as a consequence of the heavier bleeding, the mother's energies tend to be somewhat depleted." [3] Certainly, the cesarean mother who is already prone to exhaustion does not need this additional drain.

Breastfeeding is a good but *not* fail-safe method of birth control. La Leche League advises that protection from conception while breastfeeding is excellent in the first few months *if* the baby is *totally* nursed without supplemental feedings or the use of pacifier or thumb. Total breastfeeding of this magnitude is unrealistic for many of today's women who want to give their babies the best possible start, but who realize that total breastfeeding is not always possible—or, in some cases, preferable. A woman who breastfeeds her baby completely, to the exclusion of any supplemental feedings, pacification, or thumbsucking may not have much time to worry about the need for contraception—she may be so preoccupied with feeding the baby that she is too fatigued or busy to care about making love, especially if she has a "barracuda" who likes to nurse frequently and for long periods. La Leche League suggests that new mothers be fitted with a diaphragm or ask their partners to use condoms in addition to the protection of breastfeeding. Birth control pills cannot be taken by nursing women, because the hormones in them may be passed on to the baby. But this is the only method that cannot be used.

A breastfed baby may (please note the word "may") be less likely to succumb to Sudden Infant Death Syndrome (SIDS). Although there is as yet no proven cause nor any proven cure to guard against this tragedy, recent evidence suggests that the breastfed infant's chances of SIDS may be reduced.

All women are supposed to be born with a "natural" mothering instinct: the instant the mother looks at her baby, she will melt with love, caring, understanding, and know-how. This "natural" instinct is fallacious. While it may be true that all women had this instinct for preserving the species in early evolutionary stages (before childbirth became a pathological "sickness" and child care a complicated process comprehended only by "experts"), love and acceptance of the baby may not come in a divine flash. Hours, days, or even weeks may pass before the mother feels truly maternal and confident of her capabilities to care for her child. The cesarean mother who has been under general anesthesia for the birth, and/or who is kept "doped up" for days afterward and separated from her baby, is more inclined to feel a sense of detachment from the bundle presented to her as "her" baby. Breastfeeding may enhance and promote the confidence she needs to care for and love her newborn.

Cesarean mothers may be prone to difficulties in relating to their babies initially. They were not able to push the baby out by themselves, and they have been separated from their babies for hours or days. In addition, their general physical condition the first few days may make it very difficult for them to respond to their babies. There may be initial feelings of unreality or disassociation and of disbelief ("You say that this baby is mine. How do I know that it's mine?"). Being able to breastfeed her baby—something special she can do—may give her the ability to finalize her pregnancy and accept her offspring.

There are important aspects of breastfeeding which are

unique to cesarean mothers. For the cesarean mother who
anticipated a natural vaginal delivery and sharing the event
with the baby's father, there may be a sense of failure. The
mother may have felt totally uninvolved in the birth, thereby
delaying the mothering process, which further compounds her
sense of failure or guilt. Breastfeeding is something most
women *can* accomplish. Exceptions are women with renal
disease, cancer, tuberculosis, heart problems, and those who
are on certain anticoagulant drugs. Breastfeeding carries a
special, profound significance for the cesarean mother. It is
something she *can* do successfully, and it is natural, womanly,
and best for baby.

Cesarean delivery is not in itself a contraindication for
breastfeeding. But the initiation of feedings may be complicated as a result of weakness, fatigue, pain, medication, and a
lack of mobility. *It can be done.* If the mother wishes to
breastfeed, she should do so by all means. She and the baby
have nothing to lose by at least trying. They have everything
to gain. It may take two or even three weeks for the mother
to feel comfortable, confident, and relaxed while nursing.
Discouragment comes easily. Encouragement and support are
hader to come by. The cesarean mother who chooses to
breastfeed, and who sticks to it, will be a very special person.
She will be the one out of five mothers who gives birth by
cesarean, and one out of ten who breastfeeds.

The decision to breastfeed is also influenced by the father.
If he thinks there is something wrong with it, or if he is afraid
that it will require too much of the mother's time and take
attention away from himself, he may try to discourage the
mother. He is probably the type of man who is jealous of the
baby for using a part of the mother's body over which he feels
he has total control and access.

Choosing to breastfeed should not be a major decision made
with fanfare, hoopla, and nagging fears—but sometimes it is.
It is so natural and so right that it should not be the subject

of debate with entire books (and entire chapters within books) devoted to it—but it is. It should be thought of as the only right way—but it isn't. Instead of the encouragement they need, mothers may find their paths blocked by doctors, nurses, family, friends, and even the baby's father. Sometimes all the mother needs to know to overcome her hesitation is that it is best for baby, and that she has the support and encouragement of people she trusts. A tense, frustrated mother who is uncertain about breastfeeding, and who does not have positive support, may have a more negative effect on her baby—who will sense her nervousness— than a comfortable, relaxed mother who gives her baby a bottle.

Babies are very different in the way they feed. Some babies are leisurely nursers and sometimes appear uninterested in feeding. Others may be real "go-getters" and "eager beavers" (the "barracuda" type) who suck the minute the nipple reaches the mouth and who want to be fed often and for long periods of time.

Nursing does place extra nutritional demands upon the mother. If you're a nursing mother, drink at least 10 glasses of liquid a day (water, beer, milk, or juices), and try to have at least 80 grams of protein a day. Liver and greens such as spinach will also add to your iron intake, a vital nutrient for nursing mothers. Many mothers suggest keeping a thermos full of ice water or juice beside the bed at night. You won't have to get out of bed when you awaken thirsty—and you will probably be thirsty for as long as you nurse your baby.

The closeness breastfeeding affords is without equal. The benefits to the baby are tremendously important. And if the mother feels that she is a "failure" or "less womanly" because she hasn't been able to push the baby out herself, she can do something that is right and natural after all. The mother who breastfeeds does not have to justify her decision. But perhaps mothers who don't even consider it should ask themselves, "Why not?"

SOLID FOODS

Another question parents frequently ask is, When should the baby be started on solid foods? Naturally, each baby is different, and the pediatrician takes this individuality into account when advising new parents on when solid foods should be started. It is generally agreed that the newborn human infant receives little or no benefit from solid food before the sixth to eighth week of life.

Until as recently as twenty or thirty years ago, babies were not placed on solid foods at such early ages. This recent innovation seems to have started following World War II as a result of pressure exerted on pediatricians by parents who thought it a status symbol to feed their babies solid foods at earlier and earlier ages. Some pediatricians and parents now place babies on solids as early as one week! The new mother, thinking she is doing the right thing, with or without the encouragement of the pediatrician, sometimes feels very proud about how soon she gives her infant solids.

The newborn's stomach lining is not adequately prepared to ingest anything other than colostrum and breastmilk. Both contain elements that coat the lining of the baby's stomach and prepare the infant for other foods eventually. Many parents and professionals now believe that artificial feedings (formula), early solid foods, and rigid feeding schedules may account for more problems (such as colic, diarrhea, or constipation) than any other factor.

Until about the fifth month of life, the infant can obtain all substances needed to promote growth from the mother's milk. After the fifth month the infant needs additional iron—either from vitamin supplements or foods. It is interesting to note that the infant usually begins to cut teeth at about the same time. Teeth may be Nature's signal that it is now time to begin solid foods.

If the baby is fussy all the time, and the parents have tried everything in their power to calm the baby (such as frequent

holding and rocking), the pediatrician may advise supplement-
ing the infant's intake with solid foods before the fifth month.
Usually the pediatrician also advises the parents to observe
the baby for a few weeks after solid foods have been started.
If the infant seems to improve (that is, be less fussy), then
solid foods may be the answer. However, if there is no im-
provement, and the infant has been thoroughly examined to
rule out other medical causes for the fussiness, the parents
may continue or discontinue feeding the infant solids.

It is now known that the baby who grows fat on solid
food and formula is likely to become an overweight adult. If
an infant grows "fat" on breastmilk, the parents should not
be concerned, for this is "healthy" fat and will not contribute
to obesity in later life.

When to start the infant on solids is a matter for the parents
and the pediatrician to decide. If the doctor says, "Start
feeding him solids, he's not getting enough nourishment from
your milk," it's difficult for parents to argue with such advice.
The parents are apt to feel guilty and remiss in their duties
if they don't start giving the infant solid foods—and perhaps
just as guilty if they do. If your doctor recommends early
solids (at one week or one month or whenever) and you have
strong feelings about it, by all means talk to your doctor about
them. There may be special reasons for the decision. As a general rule, if the baby is breastfed at least six times within a
24-hour period, takes vitamins to ensure an adequate supply of
all nutrients (especially iron), gains weight slowly but surely,
and has at least six wet diapers per day, the baby is progressing
well and the parents should not be concerned.

The Death of Queen Jane

Queen Jane lay in labour for six days or more,
'Till the women and midwives had given her o'er:
"O if ye be friends as women should be,
Ye would send for the surgeon and bring Henry to me!"

The surgeon was sent for, he came with great speed,
King Henry arrived, and he was aggrieved,
The king held Jane's hand as he sat by her side,
"What aileth thee Janie, what aileth my bride?"

"King Henry, King Henry, if kind Henry ye be,
You'll pay heed to the doctor and set our babe free!
King Henry, my beloved, will ye do this for me?
Let them open my side to save our sweet baby!"

"Queen Jane, dearest Janie, that I'll never do,
To rip open your side would mean sure death for you!"
"Dear Henry, my husband, this I do implore:
To at least save our baby, tho I'll be no more."

The doctor gave her rich caudle,* but into death slipped she,
They pierced open her side and set the babe free.
The babe it was christened and put out to nurse,
Whilst royal Queen Janie lay cold on the earth.

Six knights and six lords bore her corpse through the grounds,
Six dukes followed after in black mourning gowns.
So black was the mourning, so black were their bands,
So black were the weapons they held in their hands.

The bells they were muffled, and mournful did play,
Whilst royal Queen Janie was buried that day.
The flower of England was laid cold in the clay,
Whilst royal King Henry came weeping away.

They mourned in the kitchen, they mourned in the hall,
But royal King Henry mourned longest of all.
"Fare thee well my beloved," he grieved his heart sore,
"The Red Rose of England shall flourish no more."

Adapted from Child ballad #170.
Jane Seymour, wife of Henry VIII, died shortly after giving
birth to Prince Edward in October of 1537. Actually, she did
not have a cesarean delivery although folk history credits her
with one. She died of childbed fever two weeks after delivery.

*Caudle: Sweetened wine

CHAPTER 15 HISTORY AND EVOLUTION OF
THE CESAREAN DELIVERY

Birth in this extraordinary manner, as described in ancient mythology and legend, was believed to confer supernatural powers and elevate the heros so born above ordinary mortals.[1]

*H*OW IS IT that we have been able to arrive at a procedure that is so safe that it is preferred to a long, complicated, or difficult vaginal delivery? If it so "good" why was it not used more often, even as recently as five or ten years ago?

The cesarean as it is performed today is the product of centuries of trial and error, experimentation, and far more failures than successes. The operation is now safe and relatively painfree. With anesthesia, antisepsis, improved surgical techniques and equipment, blood transfusions (if necessary), prenatal tests to determine fetal maturity and well-being, and advances in the care of the newborn, both mother and father can approach the delivery with confidence, knowing there is minimal risk involved and great promise of a safe delivery, comfortable recovery period, and a healthy baby.

Ask anyone where the term "cesarean section" comes from. They'll tell you that Julius Caesar was the first person to be delivered in this manner, and that we have named the operation in his honor. This belief is most assuredly untrue. Surgical delivery was known for at least one thousand years before Caesar's lifetime—although it was seldom performed on living women. *Williams Obstetrics* offers this explanation:

It has been generally asserted that Julius Caesar (100–44 B.C.) was brought into the world by this [surgical] means and obtained his name from the manner in which he was delivered (*a caeso matris utero*). . . . In the Roman law, as codified by Numa Pompilius (762–715 B.C.), it was ordered that the operation should be performed upon women dying in the last few weeks of pregnancy in hope of saving the child. This *lex regia*, as it was called at first, under the emperors became the *lex caessarea*, and the procedure itself became known as the *caesarean* operation. . . .[2]

The term probably is derived from the Latin, *partus caesareus*, from *caedere*, to cut. The term caesarean section, therefore, is really a redundancy. There is no evidence to show that Julius Caesar was thus delivered. Caesones (children delivered by section from their dead mothers) were known long before Caesar's time, and the operation was not performed on the living in Rome. Caesar's mother was alive at the time of his wars, as is proved by his letters to her.[3]

One of the earliest mythological references to the cesarean delivery is the birth of Aesculapius, historically regarded as the "god" of medicine and the son of Apollo and Coronis.[4] Variations of the tale credit either Eileitheyria, midwife to the gods at that time (1300 B.C.), or Apollo for removing the child from his mother's uterus as her body was being carried to its funeral pyre.

As expected, the one consistency I found in researching the cesarean procedure through history has been inconsistency. For example, some texts claim that the ancient Egyptians make no recorded references to this surgical method of delivery. Others, such as *Principles and Practice of Obstetrics* (1943 edition) claim:

Cesarean section on the dead woman has been done for ages, possibly even by the early Egyptians, and the operation is referred to in the myths and folklore of European races. . . . Cesarean section on the living is of more recent date, though it is more than possible that it was performed by earlier peoples. That the Jews did the operation successfully is shown by their laws. In the Mischnejoth (before 140 B.C.), the rights of twins delivered by section are gravely considered and the Talmud (400 A.D.) the law reads, "a woman need not observe the usual days of purification after abdominal delivery." "Jotze Dofan" was the name they applied to a child delivered by operation through the flank of its mother, and "Kariyath Habbeten" to the classic cesarean. . . .[5]

The lack of information about cesareans extends from the pre-Christian era to the Renaissance period. *Gynecology and Obstetrics* reports:

It will be seen, therefore, that the practice of obstetrics during the Renaissance remained much as it had been during the Greek and Roman periods with the result that, as Garrison puts it, "in normal labor, a woman had an even chance, if she did not succumb to puerperal [child-bed] fever or eclampsia; in a difficult labor she was actually butchered to death by a Sairey Gamp [midwife] of the time or one of the vagabond 'surgeons.' "[6]

The first successful cesarean section (successful in the sense that the woman lived through it) is recorded as having taken place in the year 1500. However, it was not noted until 88 years later by Caspar Bauhin, so its veracity is subject to some debate. Factual or fictionalized, this first successful cesarean took place in Singerhausen, Switzerland, where Joseph Nufer, a castrator of pigs (swine gelder) performed the operation on his wife. The Nufer family must have had some means, or at least influence in the community, for it is said that thirteen midwives were in attendance for this labor which was long, complicated, painful, and without progress. Several stone-cutters were also reported present although what they were there for is unknown. Nufer obtained permission from the authorities to do a cesarean and invited the midwives to stay. All but two left. As a swine gelder, Mr. Nufer must have been aware, however crudely and unknowingly, that sharp instruments, cleanliness, neat incisions, and suturing were essential, because the baby was safely delivered. We are told that it lived to the age of 77 and that the mother later gave birth vaginally to twins and delivered four more times after that.[7]

Other instances of cesarean section were recorded during the sixteenth century. This surgical delivery was then frequently accompanied by removal of the uterus (hysterectomy) which was deemed necessary to staunch the hemorrhaging. On the small chance that the woman survived, it's highly unlikely that she would have wanted another baby, so the hysterectomy was an extreme, but possibly welcome form of birth control. The possibility of the mother's survival was taken into account along with the grim alternatives: certain death for both, or death of the fetus by craniotomy (puncture of the skull to collapse the head, thus making it possible to remove the fetus). Champions of the cesarean procedure were often called assassins because of the extraordinarily high mortality rate.[8]

Among the outstanding events of the Renaissance was the development of cesarean section of the living woman, in the major European countries. The death rate of cesarean section at this time was almost 100 per cent. So it was quite a desperate procedure and attempted only on women who were moribund [at the point of death]. However well-intentioned the operator, the bereaved relatives always had the feeling that the unfortunate mother might have lived if she had been left alone. . . .[9]

Because of the high mortality rate, the operation was banned in Paris during the seventeenth century.

In his work "The Country Midwife's Opusculum on Vade Mecum," Percival Willughby (1597–1685) of England had this to say about cesarean section:

It hath proved unfortunate to severall, under whose hands the women have perished, and it is not used in England.

Dr. James Primrose holdeth it to bee a rash peece of work, and to do it on a living woman, a practice to be abhorred.

I therefore pass over it with silence, being unwilling to make a dreadful noise in the cares of women, or to embolden any in the works of cruelty.

Yet let mee not leave women in their sufferings comfortless, without any hope of cure, for that I beleeve this dreadful operation may, without cutting the mother's side, and womb, bee better performed, and helped, by drawing the child, if it bee living, by the feet; if it be dead, by the crochet. . . .

I therefore prefer the use of the hand before the crochet, or any other instruement whatsoever.[10]

The Italian Scipone Mercurio (1550–95?) is credited with greatly improving the knowledge of obstetrics, and is said to have revived interest in the procedure:

It was his observations on cesarean sections in France [1571] that prompted him to study under Arantius at Bologna on his return to Italy. From him, he learned much of obstetrics that bears directly on the problems of cesarean section, such as pelvic contractions. . . . He was, so far as known, the first to suggest the advisability of a cesarean operation on a living mother with a contracted pelvis . . . . His description of cesarean section is very long and detailed, but a model of clarity . . . suffice it to say that they used no anesthesia. . . . The patient was held by five strong men (or strong, courageous women) in a big canopied bed. The incision was outlined in ink first. The uterus was sponged out, as was the abdominal cavity. The abdominal wall was closed by interrupted sutures, the intestines carefully pushed away in the process. The postoperative treatment was the same as for any other form of surgery. He ends his discourse by saying, "This is enough about this new method of aiding difficult deliveries to help miserable patients."[11]

A Dutch surgeon and a contemporary of Rembrandt's, Hendrik von Roonhuyze, also advocated the cesarean section and produced a remarkable book in 1663 that contained detailed copperplate illustrations showing his method.[12]

The first successful American cesarean took place in Edom, Virginia, on January 14, 1794, when Dr. Jesse Bennet's wife was having a long and difficult labor. Dr. Bennet called in a consultant, Dr. Humphrey, whose opinion was that should a cesarean section be performed, it would most assuredly be fatal to the mother. Mrs. Bennet wished to at least save the life of her child (craniotomy being the alternative) and so insisted upon the cesarean in spite of the consultant's dire predictions.

Mrs. Bennet was placed on planks stretched across two barrels. She was held down by two Negro servants, while her sister-in-law held a lamp. The only anesthesia was a large dose of laudanum. Dr. Bennet performed the operation assisted, however condescendingly, by Dr. Humphrey. Not only did the mother survive the delivery by 36 years, but the child is said to have lived for 77 years.[13]

Another successful early American cesarean delivery took place in 1827. This operation, performed by Dr. John L.

Richmond, was done upon a kitchen table with a penknife. It is said that this mother fully recovered in 24 days.[14]

In 1879 Felkin reported witnessing a cesarean delivery in Africa. The mother was made drunk on banana wine. Then the doctor's hands and her abdomen were covered with wine. According to Felkin, the accuracy and speed with which the African doctor performed the cesarean caused him to speculate that perhaps the procedure had been known by these people for centuries.[15]

In addition to nineteenth-century developments of anesthesia and antisepsis (both unknown previously), one of the greatest advances in the cesarean delivery came in 1882 when Max Sanger developed a technique to close the uterine incision with sutures. Prior to this innovation, the uterus was always removed. With the suturing technique, removal was no longer deemed necessary.[16]

Some of today's health professionals and parents are alarmed at the rapidly growing incidence of cesarean deliveries. Depending upon one's perspective, this increase is blamed on such diverse conditions as the malpractice crisis, doctors being "knife-happy" and mercenary (an additional fee of $100 or more is charged for a cesarean), fetal monitoring (which is done routinely in many hospitals), on the use and overuse of medication and obstetrical intervention during labor, and to a host of other "causes." Before seeing this increased incidence in a totally negative light, it is important to explore several other avenues of thought.

First, take a walk through an old graveyard. How many of those headstones belong to women who died in childbirth? And those smaller markers of babies who died at birth: how many of them could have been saved if their mothers had been able to have a safe cesarean delivery?

Second, before all cesareans are written off as "unnecessary," let us ask if the *increase* in the number of cesareans will also *decrease* infant mortality, brain damage, retardation, and learning disabilities. To my knowledge, no studies have yet been undertaken to determine whether a relationship exists between the rise in frequency of cesarean deliveries and the incidence of children born with such problems as learning disabilities or brain damage. It is known that an inadequate supply of oxygen to the fetus can have deleterious physiological and neurological effects. With fetal monitoring it is now possible to determine during labor how well the fetus is doing. Should the oxygen supply be endangered, a quick, safe cesarean can be performed to overcome this potentially hazardous situation. Even if studies were begun today to determine whether a relationship between the birthing experience and (for example) learning disabilities exists, it would take a full six years or more to compile and evaluate the findings because many problems are not diagnosed until the child has entered school and is tested.

Myths, folk ballads, and old wives' tales all relate stories of women whose birth experiences included agonizing pain and often resulted in the deaths of both the mother and her baby. Surgical delivery was used only as a last resort when all other methods, potions, and incantations failed. Chances of survival for the cesarean woman were slim. It is really only in the past few decades that the cesarean procedure has become a reliable, safe alternative. The hazards, the pain, are things of the past. Yet the prospect of the cesarean delivery can still carry feelings of anguish, tension, fear, and concern. The misgivings were, until fairly recently, well-based in fact. Only now can we say farewell to them as well as to the myth, misery, and misinformation which surrounded this alternative birthing method.

CHAPTER 16 SOME CHOICES EXPECTANT PARENTS MAY WISH TO EXPLORE: A CHECKLIST

"They are going to take the baby next week."

*T*O BE SURE, it is impossible to have a baby delivered by cesarean without the skill and assistance of a medical team and modern equipment. But to say, "They are going to take the baby . . ." sounds so defeatist. "They" are not going to take the baby anywhere. The mother is going to have her baby with "their" invaluable help. Do cesarean parents have any choice in when, how, and where their babies will be born? Is it possible to make their wishes known and have them met with consideration and respect?

Unless the delivery is to take place in a hospital where the cesarean birth is already considered a birth experience in the true sense of the word, cesarean couples will need to make their preferences known. With luck and determination, they (or at least some of them) will be acted on.

A checklist of options which cesarean parents may wish to consider and discuss with their doctors and/or hospital administrators during pregnancy follows.

1. *Hospital admission.* When will it take place? Can it be arranged for the morning of the birth? Can the mother have preoperative tests (such as blood work) done on an outpatient basis a day or two before delivery so she does not have to spend the night before in the hospital?

A few hospitals already schedule important tests and interviews prior to admission or a few hours before the scheduled delivery. Coming to the hospital a few hours before the baby is born may ensure a better night's rest for the mother and will make the event seem more like a birth and less like a routine surgical procedure for the couple. In terms of dollars and cents, it probably allows a better utilization of hospital resources and may save the couple (or their insurance company or the taxpayer) the cost of an unnecessary overnight stay. Objections may be (a) the mother may not show up at the hospital in time (barring fire, flash flood, hurricane, or tornado, this objection is invalid); (b) the mother's condition cannot be monitored the night before; (c) the mother may spend the night "on the town" instead of resting quietly; (d) the mother may cheat and eat something after midnight (even in hospitals, food and water are available to the mother who wishes to "sneak" it); (e) it will cause a logjam of paperwork and preoperative procedures; and (f) admission the day before delivery is traditional.

2. *Prepping.* Why must cesarean women be prepped (shaved) of every single hair from beneath the breasts all the way around to the tailbone? Can a partial prep (no hair visible when the legs are together) be done instead?

3. *Prior knowledge of the types of medications given, their effects, and procedures performed.* These points are crucial. The mother will want to know why and what is being done to her and for her, for these things also affect her baby.

4. *Choice of anesthesia.* Unless there are medical contraindications (which the doctor will explain to the mother) may she have a voice in this decision?

5. *Father present for the birth.* Is it possible? It depends primarily on your doctor and the hospital where you have your baby. Even where hospital policies allow fathers to be present, some doctors may object. What is your hospital's policy and what are your doctor's feelings about it?

6. *Mirror.* Would you like to have one so you can see the baby's birth? Will your doctor or hospital provide one?

7. *Judgment of the infant's condition on an individual basis.*

What is the policy at your hospital? Can you make arrangements for a pediatrician to examine your baby within a short time after birth? Thus, even if the hospital has a routine of placing all cesarean babies under observation in the special care nursery for a 12- or 24-hour period, it may be possible for you to have and hold your baby within a short time.

8. *Holding and nursing the baby in the recovery room.* It is really not possible to nurse a cesarean baby within minutes after birth on the delivery table, as is done with vaginal births. Can arrangements be made to bring the baby to you within an hour or so in the recovery room?

9. *Where is the baby care unit placed?* In the delivery room, is the baby-warmer crib located where the mother can see?

10. *Will someone bring the baby to the mother within seconds or minutes after birth for viewing, examination, and admiration?*

11. *Requesting that the baby not be given supplemental feedings if the mother has decided to breastfeed.* What is the hospital policy? Are babies in the nursery routinely fed supplements?

12. *Rooming-in.* Does your hospital have rooming-in? If so, how flexible is the policy? How soon is it possible for cesarean babies?

13. *When are visiting hours for fathers?* Is he considered a "visitor" and allowed to come to the hospital only for an hour or two a day, or is he thought of as an integral family member free to visit as he wishes?

14. *If the father cannot be with you for the birth, can a significant other (such as a mother, sister, or special friend) be with you?*

15. *Is there sibling visitation?* May your older children visit you in the hospital? If so, when?

16. *What classes are available in your area for cesarean parents?* If none, is it possible to enroll in part of the regular childbirth education series, and receive supplemental instruc-

tion from the teacher? Failing that, will your obstetrician and/or a maternity nurse address your questions and supplement your information about your hospital's policies and routines?

CHAPTER 17 SUPPORTING CESAREAN PARENTS

A woman does not become pregnant to have a
vaginal delivery but to bear a healthy child.

*U*NLESS YOU ARE a cesarean
parent, or have taken the time to listen to cesarean parents
talk about their experiences, you may be unaware of the depth
of trauma many of them experience. After talking to and
corresponding with hundreds of couples across the country,
I am still often shocked and dismayed to hear their stories.
Just when I think I've heard it all, I discover that there is yet
another tale, at least as bad, if not worse, than the others. The
variety of their emotions and reactions to the emergency
cesarean is limited only by the number of parents who must
confront this situation.

SUPPORTING THE EMERGENCY CESAREAN COUPLE

The most important factor in making the emergency cesarean
delivery less emotionally traumatic and more positive is a
supportive nursing and obstetrical staff. When the attitude of
obstetricians and childbirth educators during pregnancy is to
emphasize the birth of a healthy baby rather than a vaginal
delivery, and the possibilities of a cesarean delivery are discussed openly and reassuringly, then parents can accept this

as an *alternative birthing method.* They are able to respond intelligently and without blind panic when the decision is made to do an emergency cesarean.

The announcement may also be greeted initially with a sense of relief, particularly if labor has been long and nonprogressive.

How parents are told that a cesarean is necessary influences their experience. One intelligent woman, exhausted after 16 hours of labor, was told by her doctor that he was going to "Take the baby from the top." All she could visualize was having the top of her head sawn off and the baby somehow extracted.

Ruth Allen, a registered nurse and childbirth educator, reports that "women who have been drugged with scopolamine, not knowing that a cesarean was in the offing, take a longer period of time—up to several years—to resolve their negative feelings about the experience."

When laboring couples are told may influence their reactions. The general practice is to keep them in the dark as long as possible. Not telling them makes it easier on the staff, both doctors and nurses. Couples who don't know won't ask questions, express their feelings and need a lot of time and support. They are instead, "good patients," even if unknowing ones. One father had been coaching and supporting his wife through a long labor, with lengthy contractions every two minutes. The staff knew that a cesarean was almost inevitable two or three hours in advance, but the parents were not told until the last minute. The husband said afterwards that if he had known there was a time limit, he would not have felt so discouraged. All he could see was labor going on indefinitely.

If possible, tell the couple when they are together. Offer a brief explanation of why and a simple step-by-step outline of what is to take place. The couple may not be able to take it all in, but they will appreciate your time. Let them ask questions and express their feelings to you. Except in cases of real emergencies such as *abruptio placenta,* there is time to explain. In rush cases, tell the father that you will send someone to explain as soon as possible. Above all, talk with the woman as you are caring for her. Allowing the couple to stay together while preparations are being made will give them additional time to reassure each other. If the couple are together, they can hold hands, ask questions, and talk and cry (if they feel like it) while the mother is being prepped and the catheter inserted. It is important for the staff to have a "You're okay" attitude toward the couple. Let them know that they are free to express their emotions and touch each other if they want to.

In the cesarean delivery room, it is important to emphasize the birth aspect. This is not just a routine procedure to the mother. As doctors and nurses, let us keep in mind that this is not a tumor being removed. Any and all talk should include the mother. Especially if the father cannot be present, it is our responsibility to make the mother feel involved and comfortable. We can talk with her and rejoice with her when the baby is born. She needs this support. We must constantly reassure her that she is doing well, that the baby is fine.

It will make a difference to the mother if she is able to establish eye contact (at least briefly at frequent intervals) with her obstetrician. The doctor may not have been trained to deal with emotions, but rather, how to perform a technically perfect operation on an organ. When he trained, he may have dealt only with patients who were heavily medicated and given general anesthesia. Today's philosophy of using spinal or epidural anesthesia and as little medication as possible, coupled with the assertiveness of parents who want a human, personal, warm experience is a totally different situation. More often than not, the doctor is willing to listen, and possibly to change.[1]

Parents who tell their obstetricians what they did or did not like about their experiences (rather than becoming increasingly more bitter and frustrated by holding in all their emotions) will help doctors realize what a positive difference they can make.

TRADITIONAL PREPARED CHILDBIRTH CLASSES

To truly prepare *all* couples for *any* eventuality, all prepared childbirth classes must include more than brief mention of the cesarean delivery. Any couple, regardless of how well prepared they are, how religiously they practice, or how well adjusted they are to their roles of procreators, *may* require cesarean delivery. No parent should have to face any form of childbirth unprepared.

Before the instructor can discuss the cesarean delivery in a straightforward, reassuring manner, she must feel comfortable with the topic herself. This may sound elementary, and indeed, it is. However, if the instructor feels that she does not know enough about the topic, or if she secretly feels that couples who have cesareans *are* failures, or if she fears talking about the cesarean delivery will unnecessarily scare couples, these vibrations will filter through to the class. She, too, must have a "You're okay" attitude.

A detailed and practical discussion of the preoperative procedures for a cesarean delivery should be included in all series. Certainly time should be spent talking about such physical preparations as preps, foley catheters, blood work, e.k.g.'s, fetal monitoring, or types of anesthesia. Tell the couples how long it will take for the baby to be born after the anesthesia is given. Most of them have no idea. Some think it will take hours. The couples in class tend to tune out and assume that a cesarean will happen to the couple beside them—never to them. It is important to stress that it can happen to any couple, regardless of which pregnancy this is.

It cannot be emphasized too strongly that cesareans must be mentioned throughout the entire class series, from the introductory class when the aims of the course are discussed, right through to the classes on newborn care. The odds are good that at least one couple in each series (and perhaps more) will have an emergency cesarean. If the subject is included in all classes, it becomes an alternative birthing method, rather than a catastrophe. Practical, reassuring information, presented comfortably, will be the instructor's contribution to helping all parents achieve more positive birthing experiences.

ESTABLISHING CLASSES SPECIFICALLY FOR CESAREAN PARENTS

When Ruth Allen and I met in 1974 there were no classes for cesarean parents. A few months later we established the country's first such classes. From observation, experience, and research we developed the Cesarean Birth Method, which weaves together the surgical and emotional aspects of the experience in a way that is factual and, above all, reassuring. As a result we have noticed that couples approach the delivery with confidence, have a smoother recovery, and experience many of the same happy emotions as do vaginally delivering parents. Cesarean parents as well as the professionals concerned with the birth have been quick to realize the benefits of prepared cesarean delivery, and now, slowly but surely, classes are being started throughout the country for parents whose babies will be delivered by cesarean. Childbirth organizations such as the International Childbirth Education Association and independent parents' groups are offering workshops, conferences, and seminars on the cesarean birth experience.

Instead of formal classes, interested parents and professionals may wish to begin slowly at first by holding informal "rap groups." Formal classes, funding, and/or acceptance into a large group such as ICEA or C/SEC, Inc., may come later. The group may decide that they prefer to remain independent and, perhaps, achieve a greater latitude.

For parents' groups wishing to initiate a program, it is advisable to invite the cooperation and support of at least one maternity nurse or obstetrician who works at the local hospital. (In areas where more than one hospital has maternity facilities, a person from each one should be invited.) Their assistance will benefit the group in a number of ways: (1) A professional can address technical questions, and allay any misgivings parents might have about procedures. (2) A representative from the hospital can keep couples informed of recent policy changes. Hospital policies change frequently and couples who delivered months or years before may be surprised (and, with luck, delighted) with new programs.

Setting up an exchange of information between the hospital and the consumer group is of primary importance and may facilitate implementation of the group's goals. Anything that is different is apt to be threatening. When you invite the cooperation of the local hospital in the early stages, your group may be more welcomed than one which gets going first and asks for assistance and advice later. This is not to say that the group should automatically bow to the hospital's wishes.

Even if the program is begun as an informal rap group it is important to choose a leader well-versed in group dynamics. She will not need to stimulate conversation, for once parents have introduced themselves, it is rare to find a group of cesarean couples who have difficulty talking about their experiences. Emoting about the experience will serve as a catharsis. It may be the very first occasion the parents have had to talk about their experiences with others who have shared similar ones. The presence of a nonintimidating doctor or nurse who can empathize with the parents, and help them to understand what took place and why, is also beneficial.

The role of the discussion leader will be to give each couple an opportunity to talk. Cesarean parents are prone (understandably so) to "getting up on a soap box" when talking about what happened to them. Outside their immediate circle of family and friends, never before has anyone been interested in what happened to them. Gently but surely, the discussion leader should be able to help the couples erase any negative "tapes" playing in their heads. Giving each couple time to retell their experience is imperative. Equally important is guiding the conversation to new, more positive areas.

Giving birth is one of the most profound and therefore significant events in the life of any couple. Couples who have had bad experiences (either because they did not know what to expect, or because their experiences were mishandled— however unintentionally) will carry the scars forever unless an effort is made to overcome these traumas. With the aid of others who can share their experiences, and with guides to help them understand what happened and why, they can be helped to have positive future deliveries.

People who doubt the advisability of preparing couples for cesarean birth need only listen to cesarean parents talk about their experiences. Those who have attended special classes are able to approach the next delivery with knowledge and confidence and have very different emotions from those who have not had the advantage of support and education. Good birth experiences enable parents to carry badges of confidence and knowledge. Whereas it may have been almost impossible for cesarean parents to relate tales of positive, almost poetically beautiful birth experiences, many are now able to do so—and they do so spontaneously and joyfully. They can be an inspiration to other parents to achieve goals formerly thought unattainable.

Your cesarean parents' group may also wish to encourage existing prepared childbirth programs to expand their presentations on cesarean births. Some courses do not even mention the word, much less give a detailed description of what happens, how it feels, and how to cope confidently. Or you may wish to sponsor your own series of classes. You'll need to find an effective instructor, develop a program, and bring it to the attention of interested couples.

The key to an outstanding educator for cesarean classes is empathy and technical training—not how many cesareans the instructor has had. Yes, cesarean mothers make excellent instructors. Groups that hope to establish classes should look at the applicant's credentials, caring and concern first. A sympathetic maternity nurse at a local hospital is ideal. To exclude anyone because she has not had a cesarean delivery is silly as well as discriminatory. It is also important to have a lay parent as a class assistant. She should have instruction in pregnancy, birth, and postpartum periods.

The class assistant should always be a cesarean mother. It is sometimes easier for couples to relate to an assistant, no matter how good the instructor is, partially perhaps, because the assistant is a lay person like themselves, and thus, potentially less threatening. The role of the assistant is to act as a liaison between the class and the instructor, help with questions of a nonmedical nature, and coach women who come to classes alone.

HOW TO DRAW PARTICIPANTS

A list of the names of potentially interested parents can be obtained from a number of sources. At first, it may be by word of mouth. Later, the hospital's regular prepared child-birth program may be able to submit names of couples who have delivered by cesarean. Obstetricians sometimes inform their cesarean clients of the group's existence, and leave the decision to call the group up to the individual client. The membership list will grow with time. Some classes have started with just two couples enrolled. Articles in local newspapers can help to spread the word.

WHO COMES TO CLASSES?

Classes will primarily include couples who know that they will have repeat cesareans. Some couples have attended the regular prepared childbirth series, and come to the cesarean classes to supplement what they have learned because their doctors have told them that there is a *possibility* of a cesarean delivery (for example, a breech presentation). Other couples come to classes following an emergency cesarean to learn more about what happened to them and why. Usually these parents are so traumatized that they have vowed, "Never again will I have another baby. I won't go through *that* again." It is not uncommon to find them back in class months later, pregnant, confident, and glowing all over with the anticipation of a new baby.

Couples who did not know about the classes before delivery, or who were unwilling to attend on the grounds that what they didn't know wouldn't hurt them sometimes come to classes after their babies have been born. They do not always attend the entire series; usually they attend only two or three classes.

SUGGESTED CLASS OUTLINE: THE CESAREAN BIRTH METHOD

Class One. Most couples have pre-enrolled. The instructor talks with each couple before classes start, so that she will be aware of their medical and emotional needs. She may then spend additional time, as necessary, on certain areas of interest and benefit to the group.

Upon arrival at Class One, the couples are asked to fill out a registration form, and while the father is doing this, the mother is asked to list everything she has had to eat and drink that day. (This serves not only as an introduction to Nutrition, but also helps to "break the ice.")

Couples are seated in a circle. All mothers are advised to wear slacks or jeans to classes, so that they are comfortable during the exercises. The couples introduce themselves, and tell which cesarean this is, and what their experiences were like. Among the topics the instructor should cover are:

Fetal growth and development (illustrations and visual aids are used)

Body mechanics (some of the usual discomforts of pregnancy such as backache, heartburn, and leg cramps, and how to relieve them)

Antenatal test to determine fetal growth and maturity (such as amniocentesis, estriol counts, and ultrasound) and how to prepare for them with confidence

Nutrition

Signs of labor and what to do

Braxton-Hicks contractions, their function and how to cope should they become uncomfortable

Pelvic rock

Relaxation Breathing Techniques (to relieve tension and/or physical discomfort during spontaneous labor, prenatal tests, the delivery, the postpartum period, and internal examinations)

Abdominal Tightening (to relieve gas pains)

Naturally, many couples will be apprehensive during this

first class. The classes should be as free-form as possible, allowing time for discussion—a necessary ingredient in any successful childbirth program. Often, in the first class parents express a strong fear about having an l/s·ratio done. Telling these couples what to expect and how to cope effectively is the most valuable reassurance that can be offered.

Class Two. A discussion of everything that happens from hospital admission and the attendant paperwork, to how to relieve boredom and apprehension the day before, preoperative routines, medications, how to make the administration of anesthesia easier, the actual delivery (including such information as fundal pressure and hypotension, and the recovery room period. Relaxation breathing and abdominal tightening rehearsal.

Class Three
Tour of the maternity floor, labor rooms, delivery room, recovery room, and special care nursery (this tour reinforces what has been taught in Class Two)
Explanation of each piece of equipment, and its relation to the birth process
Postpartum hospital stay (what to expect and how to cope)
Slide presentation of a cesarean birth prepared at an individual hospital. This kind of presentation further familiarizes the couples with the hospital's settings, situations, and staff. (At the hospital where I assist, a tape presentation is not used. We've found that the couples have many questions which the tape presentation would prevent us from dealing with as they arise.) By Class Three, even formerly anxious parents will probably be more confident and positive

Class Four
Postpartum discussion (caring for the infant, breastfeeding, birth control, sexual readjustment, layette needs, touching and bonding, etc.)
Two couples from the previous series are invited to discuss their experiences, and answer questions. Often these gradu-

ate parents have toddlers at home and are able to share practical tips on how to care for the toddler even though one's doctor may have warned the mother not to lift anything over 10 pounds! Class four ends with a film, "Are You Ready for the Postpartum Experience?" (available from Courter Films and Associates, R.D. 1, Box 355B, Columbia, New Jersey 07832). Diplomas and gift packs may be given out, and a party, with food and beverages provided by the class participants, will end the series on a festive note.

Sometimes an obstetrician or anesthesiologist is invited to Class Three or Four to address parents' questions. It depends upon class interest and the availability of a doctor for that particular evening.

Mothers-to-be practice relaxation breathing techniques before the close of each class.

Father participation is encouraged in all phases of the classes and the hospital period.

Audiovisual aids are important. From our experience, we have learned that detailed, graphic pictures which concentrate only on surgical technique upset couples. Photographs taken at an angle where the mother is shown as the physicians operate are much more reassuring and welcome. Just as there are negative comments on films and slides of vaginal deliveries which concentrate *only* on what the doctor sees, so too, have cesarean parents expressed distaste at seeing everything a doctor must do to perform a cesarean. Slides should emphasize the human birth aspect as well as show some of the basic operative procedures.

When fathers cannot attend classes, a significant other—a sister, mother, or friend—is always welcome. Mothers who have had cesarean deliveries many years before enjoy coming to classes with their daughters. Observers such as student nurses or instructors from other areas wishing to establish classes are welcome, providing there are only one or two in each class. The integrity of the couple's relationship with the hospital must be maintained. Too many observers may inhibit the couples, making them feel like guinea pigs.

Setting up classes may take a great deal of time and effort. Until now there has been little support and information available. As recently as five or ten years ago attitudes about prepared vaginal birth were quite different from what they are now. Today in all but the most backward areas, the advantages of prepared, shared vaginal births are widely acknowledged. The new era of regarding cesarean births in the same light of understanding and concern has just begun.

CHAPTER 18 THE WAY IT WILL BE

The experience of bearing a child is central to a woman's life. Years after the baby has been born she remembers acutely the details . . . and her feelings as the child was delivered. One can speak to any grandmother about birth and almost immediately she will begin to talk about her own labours. . . .

When women have suffered in childbirth—have felt humiliated and degraded by pain, through being the passive instruments of physical processes they could not understand—it is not only they who are affected. They carry with them through their lives the memory of this experience and by their attitudes towards child-bearing affect other women and men—not only their own daughters and sons, but many others with thom they come into contact. . . .

But when a woman has her baby happily she spreads a different spirit—a mood of gladness rather than dread and horror. . . .

It is this spirit of hope, this joy in birth as fulfilment of a man and woman's love for each other, that should be the essence of childbirth. . . .

It is childbirth with joy.[1]

The new climate of concern for cesarean families, and an understanding of their very special needs coupled with education and support, now makes it possible for cesarean parents to have experiences which embrace the essence of childbirth.

It is cesarean childbirth with confidence, empathy, dignity, and joy.

APPENDIX

BIRTH EXPERIENCES

I had three very easy vaginal deliveries and was counting on another one when in my sixth month I developed herpes. After much discussion with my ob/gyn and other doctors, I still would not accept the probability of a cesarean section. We continued our Lamaze classes and practiced the breathing techniques right to the end.

Approximately 48 hours before my surgery, we both went to see my ob/gyn who examined me, and with his colleague, found herpes lesions present. They immediately sent me for fetal X rays to determine the age and condition of the baby. The radiologist reported that the baby was ten days from term, and apparently healthy.

Over the weekend I tried to get more information about cesarean sections and the end result was some very scary stories from women who had had very unpleasant experiences with cesarean sections. This only increased my anxieties.

Finally, Monday morning arrived and I was admitted to the hospital. The anesthesiologist came up to my room to discuss the anesthesia, encouraging me to have a spinal. At first I didn't want to, but I was convinced by him to have a spinal. I was prepped and taken downstairs to the surgical suite where I said goodbye to my very supportive but nervous husband.

I was wheeled into the operating room where two nurses and the anesthesiologist were awaiting me. They scrubbed me and administered the spinal and slowly it took effect. I felt that I was being treated very much as an object rather than as a person as all this went on. Although I had sustained a good relationship with my doctor for about four years, he came into the operating room with his associate and the pediatrician and he did not once speak directly to me. I assumed this had something to do with trying to remain objective. The pediatrician acknowledged me with a nod.

I was able to observe very little due to the surgical sheets and my position, a tilted one, head being lower than feet by quite a bit. [NOTE: The table is usually tilted to the left, which may have caused this sensation.] I was amazed at how objective I became about my own body once all the feeling had left it. The sight of my own blood and the amniotic fluid passing by my head in a suction tube fascinated me. I felt quite a lot of pressure in my chest . . . I felt slightly nervous but very excited to see our baby.

Soon there was a lusty cry and they cleaned him off and wrapped him up. I only caught a glimpse of him as he was rushed upstairs to the nursery. I did not know at the time but he was very sick and was having breathing problems He was diagnosed as having either pneumonia from aspirating amniotic fluid, or hyaline membrane disease. He was very sick for about a week.

I was taken to the recovery room for a while and then back to my room. The memories are hazy from here on due to constant medications. I was very sleepy for about 48 hours but got up to be wheeled down to the nursery. The sight of our baby fighting for each breath in that incubator was quite alarming.

I was encouraged to walk up and down the halls as I slowly gained strength and was taken off the i.v. and catheter and put on a bland diet. I'm convinced that this walking was the greatest recuperative measure.

It was emotionally very hard to accept the fact of the cesarean after all the months of planning to share the birth, but the baby's illness seemed to suppress those feelings. The fact that I could not hold him was very painful, and I shed many tears over that. I had this strong feeling that if I were able to hold him all the complications would go away. Maternal omnipotence, I suppose. I was very distressed over his lack of contact with human love, warmth, skin, etc.

I had anticipated this birth as something my husband and I could share together. Naturally, I felt cheated because we were unable to accomplish this, but I do not have any negative feelings about cesarean births per se. They could be made a sharing experience, too, with a few changes.

The following are my husband's impressions:

My immediate feeling when Suzanne told me she might have our baby by cesarean was denial. I have four children by a previous marriage and I was totally left out of the birth process with all four. I was extremely excited and felt very much counted in when Suzanne told me she wanted to have our child using the Lamaze method. This meant that not only would I be present, but more than that, that I would be an active participant.

Finally during the final months of Suzanne's pregnancy, the doctor informed me that a cesarean was inevitable. I accepted the fact at this point, but was very hurt and angry— once again feeling totally put aside and left out.

We went to the hospital together and I stayed with Suzanne right up to the time she was wheeled into the operating room. My feelings at that point were very mixed up. I was afraid something might happen to Suzanne or our baby during the surgery. I was still angry about being left out, and I was very much alone.

The wait for me, during Suzanne's surgery, was very difficult. Although it took only fifty minutes, it seemed to me that I waited for a lifetime. As the time wore on, I became more nervous and anxious. Finally after about sixty-five minutes of waiting, the doctor came out and told me that we had a son and that Suzanne was fine. I was very relieved and immediately went up to the nursery while Suzanne was still in the recovery room. I met our pediatrician in the hallway outside the nursery and he informed me that Ethan had experienced some difficulty during the cesarean, and had some problems, but that he felt that everything would be all right.

I then went down to Suzanne's room and spent some time with her. Because I was not employed at the time, I had the opportunity to spend a lot of time with her during the hospital stay.

It has taken me quite a while to get over the anger of being left out of the birth experience.

I think it is very important that a couple know as much as possible, what to expect regarding cesarean birth—not only during the actual surgery, but before and after as well.

> Suzanne and Phil Hilton
> Albuquerque, N.M.

This birth was our second cesarean. With my first I was very much in the dark as to what was going to happen.

With my first I had fluid taken and checked; with this one I had a "scan or ultrasound" which was a lot nicer—for I could see the baby before it was born.

I had decided to nurse my baby, but due to my incision I bottle-fed the second one. Nursing and a cesarean operation were too much for me.

I received a spinal the first time, but it didn't take and I was "put out." This time when I had the spinal it took and I was awake for the birth of my baby. It was a strange experience. I felt nothing and was awake. Everyone was talking and the relaxed atmosphere made our baby's birth a joy. I got to see him as soon as he was born, and my husband held him until I left for the recovery room and they took the baby to the nursery.

As for me, after my operation I found the going a bit rough. It seems everything, every move, sneeze, etc., is connected and hurts. Moving is slow and you wonder if you will survive. But the next day (the second) you move a little better and a little faster. From then on you improve each day.

You should have help when you go home for at least a week. You cannot do your housework and care for your baby alone. The "around-the-clock" care of a newborn is quite demanding in its own way, and you do require rest and care. It took me about three weeks before I could handle part of the house and baby.

You must exercise after because you do have a flabby belly and must get it back in shape. It's the only way (slow).

Shirley's husband, Ron, writes:

This is the second time I was in to see a c-section baby delivered. Our first was born in June 1972. The first time I was only there for the baby being delivered. This time I was there from the first cut to the last stitch. I was in a hospital gown and face mask. I was very relaxed. My wife was awake all the time. The doctor, my wife, and all personnel were kidding and talking all the time. We were hoping for a boy and got one! I was amazed at all the cutting the doctor does before he gets to the baby, and he does not harm the baby at all. I had my camera with me and when the doctor took out the child, I got my camera ready and shot the picture, but the flash didn't work. I was amazed at how blue the baby is, and all wrinkled and doubled up. The doctor said, "Let's go baby, it's time to come out of there." The baby's hands grabbed onto one of the doctor's tools, so maybe he'll be a doctor. The doctor handed the baby to a nurse, she wrapped him in a blanket, and then handed him to me. I held him for about fifteen minutes and in that time, I showed him to my wife.

I was very alert during the whole process. I did not feel sick and was not ready to leave until the doctor did. I am very thankful we have a happy, healthy boy.

Shirley and Ron Eyrich
Temple, Pa.

Our recent family-centered cesarean delivery was an exciting birth. While I was being given the spinal, Jim was asked to wait in the corridor. He didn't realize the anesthesia and surgical preparations would take at least a half hour. After ten minutes or so, he became very anxious, fearing that the delivery was being performed without him. I was kept well-informed; although I knew he was dressed and ready, no one briefed Jim on my progress. As a result, by the time he was called in he was quite nervous and upset, but was able to relax and enjoy the delivery after he joined me.

During the operation the hospital staff gave us a great deal of support and appeared to accept my husband's presence enthusiastically. Jim seemed to have a positive effect on the atmosphere. Everyone became very excited as our child was being delivered. The enthusiastic reports of progress as Elizabeth was being delivered, to the final cheer from all that it was a girl, were very special. Jim's presence drew us all together in a very special way and helped to form an important bond between this child and her parents that continued to grow during the following months.

We were delighted to have Elizabeth cared for in the regular nursery for the first 24 hours. The rooming-in policy at the hospital allowed me to enjoy her when I was rested and comfortable, and yet I felt no pressure to provide care and companionship beyond what I felt capable of giving. By the third day, I assumed almost full care of Elizabeth, and when we left the hospital, I felt I knew her well.

We are deeply grateful to the many people who provided our family with a very wonderful start to our child's life. We hope that it will soon be possible for many couples to have the same opportunity.

Susan and James Belanger
Wellesley, Mass.

I had been told for 17 years that if I ever did conceive and carry to term, to count on a section. When I went in for a pregnancy test, I asked my doctor to do pelvimetry. At six months I repeated my request—with the same negative response. As an R.N., I know you can't really tell until the mother is in labor, the baby positioned, etc., if a section is necessary. But I felt with my history the doctor would get a pretty good idea with X rays before I went into labor.

Off to Lamaze I went (with a reluctant husband in tow). Eight weeks and $25 later, we hoped all would go well. We didn't practice much, unfortunately.

Three weeks early my water broke. Into the hospital at 12 a.m., no contractions. At 7 a.m., I was uncomfortable and antsy, but nothing definite. I was one or two centimeters dilated. By 9:30 I started to realize I was overwhelmed with pain, but there was still no pattern. None! My contractions sometimes lasted 90 seconds!

By 1:30 I was in X ray, lying on that cold, hard table with horrible back and groin pain. And a metal piece placed between my buttocks to serve as a landmark for the X ray. Other radiologists were watching outside the room, I was half-naked, and it was *awful!*

Back in the labor room, a resident came in and said a section *was* necessary. It was now 2:50 and the section was scheduled for 4 p.m.

I was prepped and shaved, had an intramuscular injection of vistaril, an antiemetic, and a tranquilizer. At 3:30 I'm wheeled off to the operating room. Well, at least the baby will be here soon and IT will be over! Into the o.r., off the cart, and onto the cold, hard operating table. And that catheter—I knew it was a garden hose and it really intensified pain.

At 4:50 in strolls the "man of the hour" (meanwhile, my husband is in the waiting room, waiting for a 4 or 4:10 phone call about his firstborn and his wife. I finally remembered to remind someone to call him and tell him of the delay. I was so angry and tired that by the time Dr. —— arrived I could have killed him! Totally unnecessary wait! It was explained that he had said a 5 p.m. section, but that the hospital had messed up.

Finally, a spinal, and at 5:04, a daughter. Two good Apgar scores; I got a fleeting glimpse of her and that was all. I was so tired, I didn't care about her as much as I "should." My cart was stopped outside the nursery to view my daughter—I hurt so bad I wanted to say, "forget it, I want a shot" but I was afraid I'd be blacklisted. (Mrs. —— is a bad mother. She cares more about herself than her baby!) Oh, well, fatigue and pain do strange things—and *anger.*

I wish I could have gotten all the anger out instead of carrying it with me two and a half years later.

Name Withheld

I had a classical incision with Christopher and was sort of willing to try to deliver vaginally the next time. There are some hospitals in this area who allow it, but knowing the risk involved I'm not sure I dare. I'd like to at least be allowed to go into labor next time because only God knows the birthday. I brought this up with my doctor and all he said was, "As long as it's elective, let's keep it that way." Naturally I worry about the baby being premature.

Susan Hemlock
Meadville, Pa.

The first time I was so ashamed I couldn't deliver normally that I wouldn't even look at anyone except my little girl. I did not even respond to my husband or doctor when they came in to recovery. Another thing that really bothered me after getting home was that I had missed enjoying and remembering my little girl's first week of life because I was so concerned about myself. Those first few days of recovery are difficult. An extra pair of hands and a body that could move easily were very welcome when the baby was in the room. I was glad for every minute my husband or anyone could spend with me. I certainly feel the husband has to pitch in more than ever in a c/sec recovery.

My second pregnancy went fine. I carried the baby low so I ended up vacuuming on my hands and knees three days before I went in. Otherwise no problems. My doctor kept me in suspense—one visit it was going to be a natural delivery, the next it could only be a c/sec. Guess this was to keep my mind off the approaching surgery. My due date was the 18th, so I entered the hospital the evening of the 13th scheduled for the next morning at 9:45. I didn't have a roommate so I got as much sleep as anyone could the night before an operation.

It was difficult going through it planned and not an emergency. They were late with the surgery because the anesthesiologist was delayed. Anyway, things got rolling about 11:30. I was so much more aware of everything. I asked many questions and requested things I knew had helped before—such as ace bandages on my legs and support stockings later.

The operation went okay. I was more aware and knew what was going on. Just before the baby was born I had terrific pains from excess oxygen under my diaphragm and they couldn't give me any pain killers until after the baby was born. I heard his weak cry and was given medication. I took one fast glance at him and that was it.

I had excellent care in recovery. I saw the baby once.

I was up on my feet a day earlier than before. Still had problems with gas. By the next afternoon I was better.

This time I was able to enjoy my baby more. I knew my recovery was on schedule so I wasn't as worried about myself.

I received no special help or counseling from the hospital. I only had one nurses aid tell me that the nursing staff was only geared to normal deliveries and they couldn't be as understanding with a section patient. She said they should all work on the surgery floor and then they would have more understanding. It is strange because it is a big hospital and they have many cesarean deliveries.

Judith Sorton
Elgin, Ill.

My particular cesarean was very traumatic. Needless to say I didn't expect the c-section. My husband and I attend Lamaze classes and were very excited about experiencing natural (as possible) childbirth. Well, after waiting 12 days past due date, I finally went into labor. I labored around 18 hours. About the time that I was 8 centimeters the doctor began thinking I might have to have a section and he discussed it with my husband. Whether he told me or not I do not know for I have no memory of labor at all. The only thing I remember was about 30 seconds in the delivery room and fighting a black mask placed overy my face. I know I was screaming like crazy—that I do remember. I briefly remember waking in the recovery room. My husband says he was there but I don't remember.

I was unable to see my baby for almost 48 hours after his birth because he was in the premature nursery for observation for two skull fractures. He also had to be resuscitated at birth. I was unable physically to get to the nursery to see him because I developed multiple complications.

This is my major trauma: not remembering the labor that brought my child into the world, and not seeing him born. Then on top of that not being able to see him for two days was shattering. I was unable to nurse him because my milk never came in because of so many drugs in the immediate postpartum period and being so sick. I am praying for a much easier time with my second child. At least then I will have something to remember.

Midge Smitthipong
Houston, Tex.

After finding out that my first baby would be born by cesarean section six days before her birth, I checked all the books I had on pregnancy and birth, only to find a few simple words on cesarean sections.

How upset I was to know so much about normal deliveries, and hardly anything about a cesarean. I have a very conscientious doctor who believes in keeping his patients fully informed with complete explanations and descriptions so I did not enter the hospital totally unaware.

I had a truly wonderful experience with a very easy recovery. I entered the hospital with a good attitude—partially I think because my mother had three cesareans and was very encouraging. My roommate had a very negative attitude. She took it as an insult or a personal punishment administered for no reason. Apparently she had been *very* frightened before from a lack of knowledge of why and what to expect.

Audrey Hanna
Old Bridge, N.J.

We had taken a course in natural childbirth and really looked forward to being together for the entire labor and birth. Unfortunately after about 12 hours of labor it was decided that my pelvic opening was just too small. Once the decision to do a cesarean was made, it really happened too quickly for us to think about what we were missing. However, we did know we wanted to be together but my husband was refused in the operating room due to administrative policy.

I was put on a stretcher flat on my back, which was very painful while still in labor, and wheeled to the operating room. I first had a slight altercation with the nurse who wheeled me down about taking my glasses off (I'm blind as a bat!). She finally agreed but I could put them on only to see the baby born and then had to take them off again. I was rather impersonally prepped. A nice anesthesiologist

administered a spinal and I was given oxygen until the baby
was born. I wish I could have at least viewed his birth via
overhead mirrors but again this was against hospital policy
in an operating room—delivery room is okay, but not in the
operating room. My husband was not even allowed in the
amphitheater.

As soon as Douglas was born, I was told I was being given
something to relax me. It made me groggy and sleepy. When
Douglas was brought to see me I was too groggy to see him
clearly. Then he was taken down to the waiting room and
shown to my husband and then put in an incubator where he
remained for 48 hours except for feedings and for the few
brief visits I had with him. I felt rather "spaced out" for
about 48 hours. I was excited about the baby but didn't
really have the ambition to ask if I could see him. Fortunately he was brought to me for about a 2-minute visit about
7 hours after he was born. I still didn't have the ambition to
ask to see him the next day but he was brought in again for
a 2-minute visit the forenoon. My husband and I still had not
been able to see him together. That afternoon I came down
with a fever. He was not brought to me again nor did I ask
till the next day.

I had amnioitis. (I had ruptured membranes about 6 days
before he was born.) Consequently, I was unable to touch
my baby until 3 days later. They did allow my husband to
feed him (I didn't breastfeed) in my room as long as I didn't
touch him. I also had to live on i.v.'s until 4 days after he was
born. I guess I really didn't feel like eating anyway. I still
felt pretty spaced out during my hospital stay. The doctor
attributed it to all the medication I was given for infection.
Next time I'd like to feel a little more in touch with reality.
I was also refused to shower or even wash my hair. That was
horrible.

The next time, my husband and I would like to go to the
hospital the day of the cesarean. We'd like to be together in
the operating room. I don't want any medication that will

make me feel groggy or spaced out. We'd like to see our baby together alone after the operation. We would like to make it more comfortable and meaningful the next time.

Priscilla and Craig Sinclair
Bristol, N.H.

I had a c-section but I did not know that I was going to have one until just before I went into the delivery room. I had a breech delivery. Also, I had the gas pains and consequently had my stomach pumped for a day plus i.v. I don't know how I got or kept my courage to nurse my boy, but I guess it was sheer determination. My arm sure hurt holding him and the i.v. in it!

Janet Wagner
Archbold, O.

From what I read in the [C/SEC] newsletter, my section was "old-fashioned"—I was put to sleep, cut in the classical way, didn't see husband or baby till hours after the operation. The reason for my section was because my pelvis is too small so I guess my future baby(s) will be delivered that way, too. But knowing more about it now, possibly I can change my doctor's (and hospital's) minds a little and maybe let me be awake. The gas pains from the anesthesia afterwards were worse than the incision discomfort.

Sandy Sagala
Erie, Pa.

I have just had my second c-section and it was worse than the first. I went to the library in Lancaster and couldn't find even the word cesarean in the files. Talk about discouragement! I thought it was just in Lancaster but when I went to Philadelphia to visit my parents, it was the same. Only one book in the whole library had a small, 1½-page, and not very detailed description of a c-section.

Linda McGlone
Levittown, Pa.

We went to natural childbirth classes and were prepared to have our baby natural. After 27 hours of labor we were told that I could not deliver naturally. We both felt really let down after working all those hours. But my second thoughts were that I was really relieved because I was so tired. Pat stayed with me and helped me through everything, and I had a wonderful doctor who really helped, too. When I knew Pat could be with me in the operating room I was really glad. The doctor wanted me to be awake for the birth but I was so tired and exhausted and I didn't know exactly what was going to happen so I wanted to be put asleep. I didn't feel I could take much more. As I was falling asleep, Pat talked to me and held my hand. Just knowing he was going to be there, I was not afraid.

When they took me to my room he was there and told me all about the birth of our daughter. He was so excited and happy. He said he wished he'd taken more pictures, but he was too interested in watching the birth of our baby. He told me if he was offered a trip around the world free, all expenses paid, or the chance to watch the birth of a baby, he would want to see the baby being born.

When I came home, Pat, my mother and mother-in-law were there to help. For the first two weeks I couldn't do very much. It was such a struggle just to stand up. After the first two weeks, I started to feel a lot better.

If you can have a baby normally, that would be wonderful,

but if you can't sharing a cesarean birth can be just as wonderful.

Debbie's husband, Pat, writes:

We had prepared for a natural birth. When the doctor said a cesarean section would have to be done I felt disappointed. She had worked so many hours in the labor room. I was nervous and upset.

Dr. —— explained everything he was going to do during the operation while we were getting into our green gowns. While putting on the gown the anesthesiologist asked me if I was a medical student. Dr. —— said no, I was the husband and was going to watch the birth of our baby. That made me feel good and I realized I was really a part of this great experience. Having a wonderful doctor like Dr. ——, who explains everything to you made a big difference. I felt secure in his judgment.

During the operation I was nervous, but I really enjoyed it. It was such a thrill, and to hear her first cry, I was overwhelmed with joy. She was so beautiful.

Right after Melissa was born Dr. —— asked me if I wanted to hold her, but I was so excited I felt I'd better not. The next child I will want to hold and take a lot more pictures. I also want to have a tape recorder to record the sounds of our baby's first cry.

When we went home I was glad to do things for Deb, after all she had to go through for us. I told her I would do anything for her, but when she was better I got tired of doing dishes, washing, and cleaning, and I let her start to do those again by herself.

It was wonderful that I could be with her, help her, and share with her this very hard but wonderful experience. It has made us so much closer.

Debra and Patrick Boylan
Leesport, Pa.

At present, I'm more determined in my pursuit of the medical phenomenon of my c-section and what went wrong. The gynecologists I see here (three in one office) insist a vaginal delivery would be too risky, if I do have a second pregnancy. However, now that I'm more emotionally clear from the trauma, I'm going back for another review of my case, and I intend to visit a specialist up at Stanford who was recently highly recommended to me.

As I understand it, my three-day labor was due to uterine inertia resulting from poor muscle pressure in the pelvis. The baby was posterior and large (9 pounds, 3 ounces). The pain and discomfort registered in my rectum and lower back. This continued long after my water broke and labor was induced. X rays also revealed that my pelvis was wide enough.

By the time they operated, I had only dilated to 6 cms. And after surgery as I was beginning to sort out all that had taken place, the doctor tells me it's a good thing they operated when they did because my uterine wall was "paper thin" and readily admitted that the "facts" just don't add up.

Amy Krupski
Pacific Grove, Calif.

I went in for emergency surgery at 5 p.m. I was lonely and scared during the prep and really had to fight to keep the tears back. They let me see my husband before going in and my fears just tumbled out. I was frightened on the operating table as my doctor hadn't arrived. The only reason I managed to stay calm was because the scrub technician talked to me. I saw someone insert the i.v. and the next thing I knew I was in pain in the recovery room. When I came around (I had general) I was in such pain I thought I was still in labor. I was having hard contractions when they put me under and so I thought I still had the baby. Every [after-birth] contraction tore at me and the nurse kept pushing on my stomach and I kept passing out. My only fear is the recovery room. I wanted my husband just to be there.

But once I got up to my room, everything was fine—except for not getting to hold my baby. But after the recovery room they wheeled me to the nursery to see my Heather Christine. My husband was there. He never left the window from the time she was born to then. He watched over her while I couldn't.

The staff was wonderful and took out the i.v. and catheter at my request at 6 a.m. the next day. I walked and walked. It felt good to have a shower and get my own nightie on. I believe the hospital tried very hard to make me happy and comfortable.

I think the important thing in my speedy recovery was my determination to get up and get clean. I didn't care how much it hurt—I walked. I walked down to see my baby, I walked everywhere. The nurses threatened to tie me down. I had a wonderful recovery and was home in 2½ days.

I have so many questions. I do not understand the operation. Three months later I still wake up with nightmares. There are many things I'd like to do differently the next time. But I'm thankful for my doctor and the hospital for their efforts in helping me.

Brenda Kent
San Jose, Calif.

My husband and I had participated in prepared childbirth classes and concentrated on our breathing and relaxation routines for a vaginal delivery—though we knew that due to my small pelvis, I was always a potential cesarean mother. The classes covered various analgesics and types of anesthesia, as well as cesarean births. We also took a hospital-encouraged predelivery visit to the labor and delivery rooms to help us get acclimated, although we weren't able to visit the operating room. We smothered our nurse-guide with questions, so in the end we felt we were modestly prepared for either method of delivery. We also knew that due to our hospital's open policy, my husband would remain with me in either case.

Labor for me ended up to be long, painful, and fruitless—lasting 12 hours at home and 10 in the hospital. Toward the end, my cervix stopped dilating at 7 cm. and never reached the delivery goal of 10 cm. Although my mind was a bit cloudy with Demerol, I do remember having a very serious mental discussion with myself as to whether it was all worth it. When the doctor decided on a c-section as the best solution for delivering the baby, my husband said my first words were, "Thank God!" The actual operation from the first incision to the baby's delivery (it was a boy) to closure of the incision with several layers of stitches took less than one hour. Because of a cesarean rather than a vaginal delivery, Kevin's head was hardly molded at all, and he arrived round and beautiful— all 8 pounds, 9 ounces of him. (I decided it *was* worth it). Since I had a spinal which took away all of my pain, I can remember chatting happily with the doctor about a new book on the market and my husband's work while the doctor completed the stitches. I had been completely awake during the operation but was unable to watch because of a cloth screen in front of my head; but, because he was there, my husband was able to describe Kevin's first moments of life and to take pictures of his birth.

My physical recovery was very smooth. Having had the spinal, I was asked to remain lying horizontal for 8 hours. But after that interval I shocked the nurses by getting up and going to the bathroom unassisted. (Actually, I thought I *did* have to get up by myself. Never having been in a hospital before, it never occurred to me to ask for a bedpan. I did experience pain after delivery, but it was less than the gas pains I felt when my intestines expanded to their normal position and filled with air. For several days I walked around slightly bent over from the unrealistic fear that standing straight would stretch open my incision—not thinking that I was straight when lying down. I also nursed Kevin, although for a day or two, I was more comfortable lying on my side to nurse rather than sitting upright. So, in four days I was ready to go home.

My birth experience doesn't end with going home, however, for nine days later I was back in the hospital with a pelvic infection spreading from my cervix, fallopian tubes, and abdomen. Five days of intravenous antibiotics took care of the infection, but having to leave Kevin was heartbreaking. Luckily, John's mother was able to stay with Kevin, and he happily (and unfortunately) drank formula until I could return and breastfeed him.

Right now I hardly think about my incision. It is only a small horizontal smile (called a "bikini cut") below my pubic hair line and will hardly show in time. I think much of my ability to cope with having a baby surgically and its aftermath is due to both my doctor and my own philosophy. My doctor was always open and "up front" about a possible cesarean delivery and thus helped me to prepare myself mentally many months before I went into labor. When the decision had to be made, I immediately understood and coped with it. I also realize that the most important goals of childbirth are life and health. Since an extended labor might have ended in a burst uterus for me or a damaged brain for my baby, I am most grateful that a cesarean delivery could provide both of us with a healthy birth.

On the other hand, looking back on our class preparation, I can't help but feel frustrated and bitter. The classes understandably emphasized techniques and postnatal exercises for natural childbirth since they would be proper for 90 percent of the couples attending. Cesarean births were covered, but only as a part of a section on atypical (one could almost read "abnormal") births, and then only briefly. That left me as a cesarean mother excluded from the norm. Also, the classes in my eyes brainwashed my husband and me into a definition of a "shared" childbirth as one in which we together relaxed, breathed, pushed, and delivered the baby—as though this were the only way to share, and no other.

We will always recommend the prepared childbirth classes to prospective parents, since we found them informative, practical, and encouraging of a special closeness between husband and wife. However, I think potential cesarean couples and prepared childbirth classes should switch from sharing by "doing" to more of an emphasis on sharing a healthy and happy birth for both mother and child, no matter how. Such a goal, I think should be much more satisfying than all the breathing techniques one could ever learn.

Her husband writes:

From the standpoint of psychological letdown at not having a natural delivery, I was luckier than most. Somehow, in the back of my mind throughout the entire pregnancy, I had the feeling a c-section would be required. That, plus 10 hours of extremely difficult labor for Connie, made the doctor's decision to operate easier to handle—in fact, it was a welcome decision to both of us.

The actual operation was a snap—from my viewpoint at least. Other than the usual run of high school cancer films and the natural delivery films from our class (discounting, of course, Marcus Welby, Medical Center, Dr. Kildare, etc.) I had never witnessed a major operation before. I definitely had my doubts about whether I could watch or not. In actual fact, it didn't faze me in the least. Whether it was the confidence I had in Dr. ——, or the 20 hours I had been awake, I don't know. I was physically and emotionally shocked when the doctor reached in and pulled Kevin out. (Wow, there really *was* a baby in there!) It was something I wouldn't have missed for the world—and something I don't intend to miss the next time around.

Names Withheld

SUGGESTED READING

PREGNANCY

Birth
Catherine Milinaire
Harmony Books

The Cultural Warping of Childbirth
Doris Haire
ICEA Supplies Center
P.O. Box 70258
Seattle, Wa. 98107

Pregnant Patients Bill of Rights
(One copy free with stamped, self-addressed envelope)
Committee on Patients Rights
Box 1900
New York, New York 10001

A Season To Be Born
Suzanne Arms & John Arms
Harper & Row

Yoga for New Parents
Ferris Urbanowski
Harper's Magazine Press

The Experience of Childbirth
Sheila Kitzinger
Penguin Books

Six Practical Lessons for an Easier Childbirth
Elisabeth Bing
Bantam Books

NUTRITION

The Complete Handbook of Nutrition
Gary & Steve Null
Dell Publishing Company

Let's Get Well
Let's Have Healthy Children
Adele Davis
Signet Books

POSTPARTUM EXPERIENCE

Touching
Ashley Montague
Harper & Row

What Now?
Mary Lous Rozdilsky and Barbara Banet
Charles Scribner's Sons

GENERAL

Our Bodies, Our Selves
Boston Women's Health Book Collective
Simon & Schuster

FOR PROFESSIONALS

Communications: Dimensions in Childbirth Education
Margot Edwards, R.N.
ICEA Supplies Center
P.O. Box 70258
Seattle, Wa. 98107

Maternal-Infant Bonding
Marshall H. Klaus, M.D., and John H. Kennell
C.V. Mosby Company
St. Louis, Missouri

ORGANIZATIONS

C/SEC, Inc.
Patricia Erickson, Membership Chairperson
23 Cedar Street
Cambridge, Massachusetts 02140

C/SEC, Inc.'s philosophies and goals focus exclusively on cesarean deliveries; and activities and publications are geared to improving the overall pregnancy, birth, and postpartum experiences of cesarean families. For membership information and/or a list of organizations in your area, send a stamped, self-addressed envelope to C/SEC, Inc.

International Childbirth Education Association (ICEA)
Mrs. Charles H. Tadge, Membership Chairperson
1819 Sheridan Road
South Euclid, Ohio 44121

ICEA is composed of individuals and groups, both laypersons and health-care professionals, whose goals and membership encompass a wide variety of disciplines, all dedicated to furthering and promoting more satisfying birth experiences for *all* parents; and to fostering better parent-child relationships. ICEA studies and disseminates knowledge concerning family-centered maternity and child care. The supplies center offers members the most recent literature for laypersons and professionals. International and regional conferences and the intraorganization publications are excellent resources exchanges.

La Leche League International
9616 Minneapolis Avenue
Franklin Park, Illinois 60131

Both a resources exchange and support organization for nursing mothers. La Leche offers publications, seminars, and community groups.

Nurses' Association of the American College of Obstetricians and Gynecologists (NAACOG)
One East Wacker Drive
Chicago, Illinois 60131

NAACOG is an organization of and for obstetric, gynecologic, and neonatal nurses. The *JOGN Journal,* published bimonthly, and NAACOG's seminars are excellent sources of up-to-date information for the practicing nursing professional.

NOTES

CHAPTER 2, INDICATIONS

1. Myles, Margaret M., *Textbook for Midwives* (Edinburgh and London: Churchill and Livingston, 1972), p. 227.

CHAPTER 3, PREGNANCY

1. Editors of Consumer Reports, *The Medicine Show*, rev. ed. (Mt. Vernon, N.Y.: Consumers Union, 1971), pp. 184-5.
2. Milinaire, Catherine, *Birth* (New York: Harmony Books, 1974), p. 51.

CHAPTER 6, SIGNS OF LABOR

1. Hellman, Louis M., and Jack A. Pritchard, *Williams Obstetrics*, 14th ed. (New York: Appleton-Century-Crofts, 1971), p. 936. The actual incidence of uterine rupture is difficult to determine "but it is probably between 1 in 1,000 and 1 in 1,500 births. . . ."
2. The 5 percent incidence is based on the author's 1976 conversations with two British midwives. The Fourteenth Edition of *Williams Obstetrics* (1971), ibid., states that "figures for England and Wales and for the Netherlands are 2.7 per cent and 1.25 per cent, respectively."

CHAPTER 8, BIRTHDAY!

1. From an address given by Ruth Allen, R.N., at the South Shore Hospital (South Weymouth, Massachusetts) Childbirth Seminar, November 22, 1975, unpublished.

CHAPTER 10, CONTROVERSY

1. *Time* Magazine, "Malpractice: Rx for a Crisis" (New York: Time, Inc., June 16, 1975), p. 49.
2. Letter dated January 20, 1976, from T. Berry Brazelton, M.D., Cambridge, Mass., to the author.

3. Letter dated February 6, 1976, from J. Robert McTammany, M.D., of Reading, Pa., to the author.

4. Letter dated February 3, 1976, from Judith Gundersen, R.N., Coordinator of Parent Education, Boston Hospital for Women, to Elizabeth Caswell, R.N., Director of Parent Education and Maternity Coordinator, South Shore Hospital, South Weymouth, Ma.

CHAPTER 14, TOUCHING AND BONDING AND THE ADVANTAGES OF BREASTFEEDING

1. Montague, Ashley, *Touching* (New York: Perennial Library, Harper & Row, 1972; copyright 1971, Columbia University Press), p. 65, pp. 75-78, *passim.*

2. Ibid., p. 91, p. 95, p. 138, *passim.*

3. Ibid., p. 53.

CHAPTER 15, HISTORY AND EVOLUTION

1. Hellman, Louis M., and Jack A. Pritchard, *Williams Obstetrics,* 14th ed. (New York: Appleton-Century-Crofts, 1971). p. 1164.

2. Eastman, Nicholson J., and Louis M. Hellman, *Williams Obstetrics,* 12th ed. (New York: Appleton-Century-Crofts, Inc., 1961), p. 1179.

3. De Lee, Joseph B., M.D., and J. P. Greenhill, M.D., *Principles and Practice of Obstetrics,* 8th ed. (Philadelphia and London: W. B. Saunders Company, 1943), p. 1011.

4. Jameson, Edwin M., M.D., *Gynecology and Obstetrics* (New York: Hafner Publishing Company, 1962), p. 25.

5. De Lee and Greenhill, op. cit., p. 1011.

6. Jameson, op. cit., p. 41.

7. Cianfrani, Theodore, M.D., *A Short History of Obstetrics and Gynecology* (Springfield, Ill.: Charles C Thomas, 1960), pp. 359-61.

8. Ibid., p. 361.

9. Op. cit., p. 131.

10. Cloud, I. G., M.D., "Cesarean Section on the Dead and Moribund" (New York: *Journal of the American College of Obstetricians and Gynecologists,* July, 1960), p. 30.

11. Cianfrani, op. cit., pp. 150-151.

12. Cianfrani, op. cit., p. 171.

13. Cianfrani, op. cit., p. 264 with additional details from a letter dated March 18, 1976, from Vance Watt, M.D., of Thomasville, Georgia, to the author.

14. Cianfrani, op. cit., p. 361.

15. De Lee and Greenhill, op. cit., p. 1011.

16. Speert, Harold, M.D., *Obstetric and Gynecologic Milestones* (New York: The Macmillan Company, 1958), p. 594.

CHAPTER 17, SUPPORTING CESAREAN PARENTS

1. From an address by Ruth Allen, R.N., given at the Childbirth Education Association of Erie (Pa.) Sharing Seminar, May 1, 1976, unpublished.

CHAPTER 18, THE WAY IT WILL BE

1. Kitzinger, Sheila, *The Experience of Childbirth* (Baltimore: Penguin Books, Inc., 1962-1972), pp. 17-18.

INDEX

9/24/82

Cesarean-
was quick operation - many jokes
Alex very sleepy baby for days
in hospital. Liked H_2O a lot.

Felt very good 2nd day - walked,
catheter + IV with antibiotics + pitocin
were out-

Contractions very hard with nursing
was given Demerol until 12PM 9/24
for pain

Epidural numbed from breast down

Tugging during operation pant

Diet liquid, mostly cuz gas can
occur

Very tired as days progress

staples

Visit from Austen - exciting -
present - rattle - very concerned.

TO DO

① type notes for cesarean class .

② mk relaxation tapes

allu austen $20
                  ‖
1.25 $10
  8
———→
$10.00
  6
75   ———
8/ $16.00
6.00   30 → $6.00

$16 3/
   48
   ×/10 $72
     56 →
       79